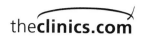
theclinics.com

OTOLARYNGOLOGIC CLINICS OF NORTH AMERICA

Advanced Techniques in Rhinology

GUEST EDITORS
Martin J. Citardi, MD, FACS
and Pete S. Batra, MD

June 2006 • Volume 39 • Number 3

SAUNDERS

An Imprint of Elsevier, Inc.
PHILADELPHIA   LONDON   TORONTO   MONTREAL   SYDNEY   TOKYO

W.B. SAUNDERS COMPANY
A Division of Elsevier Inc.

1600 John F. Kennedy Boulevard, Suite 1800, Philadelphia, PA 19103–2899

http://www.theclinics.com

THE OTOLARYNGOLOGIC CLINICS   Volume 39, Number 3
OF NORTH AMERICA   ISSN 0030–6665
June 2006   ISBN 1-4160-3587-7
Editor: Joanne Husovski

Reprints. For copies of 100 or more, of articles in this publication, please contact the Commercial Reprints Department, Elsevier Inc., 360 Park Avenue South, New York, New York 10010-1710. Tel. (212) 633-3813; Fax: (212) 462-1935; email: reprints@elsevier.com

The Otolaryngologic Clinics of North America (ISSN 0030–6665) is published bimonthly by W.B. Saunders, 360 Park Avenue South, New York, NY 10010-1710. Months of publication are February, April, June, August, October, and December. Business and Editorial Offices: 1600 John F. Kennedy Blvd., Suite 1800, Philadelphia, PA 19103-2899. Accounting and Circulation Offices: 6277 Sea Harbor Drive, Orlando, FL 32887-4800. Periodicals postage paid at New York, NY and additional mailing offices. Subscription price is $205.00 per year (US individuals), $370.00 per year (US institutions), $100.00 per year (US student/resident), $270.00 per year (Canadian individuals), $455.00 per year (Canadian institutions), $285.00 per year (international individuals), $455.00 per year (international institutions), $145.00 per year (international & Canadian student/resident). Foreign air speed delivery is included in all *Clinics*' subscription prices. All prices are subject to change without notice. **POSTMASTER:** Send address changes to *The Otolaryngologic Clinics of North America*, Elsevier Periodicals Customer Service, 6277 Sea Harbor Drive, Orlando, FL 32887-4800. **Customer Service: 1-800-654-2452 (US). From outside the US, call 407-345-4000.**

The Otolaryngologic Clinics of North America is also published in Spanish by McGraw-Hill Interamericana Editores S.A., P.O. Box 5-237, 06500 Mexico D.F., Mexico.

The Otolaryngologic Clinics of North America is covered in *Index Medicus, Current Contents/Clinical Medicine, Excerpta Medica, BIOSIS, Science Citation Index,* and *ISI/BIOMED.*

Printed in the United States of America.

GUEST EDITORS

MARTIN J. CITARDI, MD, FACS, Head, Section of Nasal and Sinus Disorders, The Cleveland Clinic Head and Neck Institute, Cleveland, Ohio

PETE S. BATRA, MD, Assistant Professor of Surgery, Section of Nasal and Sinus Disorders, The Cleveland Clinic Head and Neck Institute, Cleveland, Ohio

CONTRIBUTORS

NAFI AYGUN, MD, Assistant Professor, Neuroradiology Division, Johns Hopkins Medical Institutions, Baltimore, Maryland

PETE S. BATRA, MD, Assistant Professor of Surgery, Section of Nasal and Sinus Disorders, The Cleveland Clinic Head and Neck Institute, Cleveland, Ohio

DANIEL G. BECKER, MD, FACS, Clinical Associate Professor and Director, Division of Facial Plastic Surgery, Department of Otolaryngology, University of Pennsylvania Medical Center, Philadelphia, Pennsylvania; Clinical Associate Professor, University of Virginia Medical Center, Charlottesville, Virginia

SAMUEL S. BECKER, MD, Resident, University of Virginia Medical Center, Charlottesville, Virginia

WILLIAM E. BOLGER, MD, FACS, Professor of Surgery, Department of Otolaryngology, Uniformed Services University of the Health Sciences, Bethesda, Maryland

MARTIN J. CITARDI, MD, FACS, Head, Section of Nasal and Sinus Disorders, The Cleveland Clinic Head and Neck Institute, Cleveland, Ohio

NOAM A. COHEN, MD, PhD, Assistant Professor, Division of Rhinology, Department of Otorhinolaryngology–Head and Neck Surgery, University of Pennsylvania School of Medicine, Philadelphia, Pennsylvania

ROBERT ELLER, MD, American Institute for Voice and Ear Care and The Graduate Institute, Philadelphia, Pennsylvania

PETER H. HWANG, MD, Associate Professor, Department of Otolaryngology–Head and Neck Surgery, Stanford University, Palo Alto, California

DAVID W. KENNEDY, MD, Professor and Chief, Division of Rhinology, Department of Otorhinolaryngology–Head and Neck Surgery, and Vice Dean, University of Pennsylvania School of Medicine, Philadelphia, Pennsylvania

P. DANIEL KNOTT, MD, The Cleveland Clinic Head and Neck Institute, Cleveland, Ohio

FREDERICK A. KUHN, MD, Director, Georgia Nasal & Sinus Institute, Savannah, Georgia; Adjunct Professor, Department of Otolaryngology, University of North Carolina, Chapel Hill, North Carolina

JERN-LIN LEONG, FRCS (Glasg), Associate Consultant, Department of Otolaryngology, Singapore General Hospital, Singapore, Republic of Singapore

HOWARD L. LEVINE, MD, Cleveland Nasal-Sinus & Sleep Center, Cleveland, Ohio; Marymount Outpatient Care Center, Marymount Hospital, Garfield Heights, Ohio; Adjunct Staff, The Cleveland Clinic Head and Neck Institute, Cleveland, Ohio

CHRISTOPHER T. MELROY, MD, Chief Resident, Department of Otolaryngology–Head and Neck Surgery, University of North Carolina Hospitals, Chapel Hill, North Carolina

RALPH METSON, MD, Professor, Department of Otology and Laryngology, Harvard Medical School; Department of Otolaryngology, Massachusetts Eye and Ear Infirmary, Boston, Massachusetts

RICHARD R. ORLANDI, MD, Associate Professor, Division of Otolaryngology–Head and Neck Surgery; Associate Director, Center for Therapeutic Biomaterials, The University of Utah, Salt Lake City, Utah

SHIRLEY S.N. PIGNATARI, MD, Professor and Head, Division of Pediatric Otorhinolaryngology, Federal University of São Paulo, Paulista School of Medicine; Chief, Pediatric Otolaryngologic Division, São Paulo ENT Center, Hospital Professor Edmundo Vasconcelos, São Paulo, Brazil

STEVEN D. PLETCHER, MD, Department of Otolaryngology, Massachusetts Eye and Ear Infirmary, Boston, Massachusetts

RODNEY J. SCHLOSSER, MD, Associate Professor and Director of Rhinology and Sinus Surgery, Department of Otolaryngology–Head and Neck Surgery, Medical University of South Carolina, Charleston, South Carolina

BRENT A. SENIOR, MD, Associate Professor and Chief of Rhinology, Allergy, and Sinus Surgery, Department of Otolaryngology–Head and Neck Surgery, University of North Carolina Hospitals, Chapel Hill, North Carolina

DHARAMBIR S. SETHI, MD, FRCSEd, Senior Consultant, Department of Otolaryngology, Singapore General Hospital, Singapore, Republic of Singapore

MICHAEL SILLERS, MD, Alabama Nasal and Sinus Center, Birmingham, Alabama

ALDO CASSOL STAMM, MD, Professor, Department of Otorhinolaryngology, Head and Neck Surgery, Federal University of São Paulo, Paulista School of Medicine; Director, São Paulo ENT Center, Hospital Professor Edmundo Vasconcelos, São Paulo, Brazil

EDUARDO VELLUTINI, MD, Director of the DFV Neuro; Director, Department of Neurosurgery, Hospital Oswaldo Cruz, São Paulo, Brazil

P.J. WORMALD, MD, FRACS, FCS (SA), FRCS, MBChB, Professor, Department of Surgery–Otolaryngology, Head & Neck Surgery, The Queen Elizabeth Hospital, Adelaide and Flinders Universities, Woodville, South Australia, Australia

S. JAMES ZINREICH, MD, Professor, Radiology, Otolaryngology, Head and Neck Surgery, Johns Hopkins Medical Institutions, Baltimore, Maryland.

CONTENTS

Radiologic imaging is an essential part of the presurgical evaluation
of patients with sinusitis and of the monitoring of difficult-to-treat,
recurrent, and postsurgical disease. In patients with noninflammatory sinus pathology and those who "baffle" clinical diagnosis, imaging is extremely helpful in differentiating the various pathological
entities and determining the extent of disease. Computerized tomography (CT), when deemed clinically necessary, is the current modality of choice to evaluate sinusitis. CT's ability to display bone,
mucosa, and air makes it a perfect tool for imaging of the paranasal
sinuses. The fine bony architecture of the nasal cavity and the paranasal sinus drainage pathways are depicted accurately with CT
examination.

Patients with recurrent chronic sinusitis after prior surgical intervention pose a particular challenge to the otorhinolaryngologist.
Establishing a correct diagnosis is the first step. Although primary
chronic rhinosinusitis is typically a medical disease, postsurgical
persistent disease may result directly from iatrogenic causes, requiring early surgical revision. Even in this setting, however, proper
preoperative medical therapy is essential. When the decision to
undergo revision surgery is made, the patient and the physician
need to comprehend the rigorous and prolonged schedule of postoperative care and débridements that may be required for long-
term success. Medical management and endoscopic surveillance
postoperatively is continued until a stable cavity is achieved.

strategies, surgical techniques, and outcomes data for the minimally invasive endoscopic resection.

Transnasal endoscopic-assisted techniques to the clivus region can be safe and effective. Endoscopic-assisted approaches provide improved visualization and are a superior alternative to open surgical approaches in most cases. Nevertheless, problems such as infection, CSF leakage, and difficulty controlling intradural bleeding still remain. Surgeons must always remember that, although high technology such as endoscopes, image-guided surgery systems, imaging studies, and advanced anesthetic drugs were essential for the development and improvement of the skull base surgery, the success of this type of surgery depends on perfect knowledge of the anatomy, intense endoscopic surgery training, and a multidisciplinary partnership.

FORTHCOMING ISSUES

RECENT ISSUES

The Clinics are now available online!

Access your subscription at
www.theclinics.com

Otolaryngol Clin N Am
39 (2006) xiii–xiv

OTOLARYNGOLOGIC
CLINICS
OF NORTH AMERICA

Preface

Advanced Techniques in Rhinology

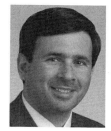 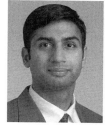

Martin J. Citardi, MD, FACS   Pete S. Batra, MD
Guest Editors

Over the past decade, rhinology has experienced a period characterized by numerous innovations. Most, but not all, of these developments have been related to strategies for endoscopic sinus surgery. In its original form, endoscopic sinus surgery was conceived as a method to treat refractory inflammatory disease of the paranasal sinuses through improving sinus ventilation. Over the years, endoscopic techniques have become increasingly sophisticated and the indications for endoscopic approaches have grown.

Various factors have catalyzed a shift in the management of diseases of the paranasal sinuses. Otorhinolaryngologists have embraced the trend for minimally invasive surgery and have developed endoscopic techniques for conditions that previously would have required more extensive "open" procedures. Technologic developments have also had a dramatic impact. Diagnostic imaging supports more accurate and precise diagnosis. Better instruments designed to meet the needs of the endoscopic surgeon have been introduced. Powered instrumentation, including drills, has been significantly improved. Computer-aided surgery serves as a platform for preoperative planning and intraoperative surgical navigation. Thus, the tools available to the otorhinolaryngologist are much more sophisticated today than even a few years ago.

This issue of *Otolaryngologic Clinics of North America* summarizes some of the latest developments in surgical rhinology. Of course, including all aspects of the rapidly growing domain of rhinology is simply not feasible; instead, this issue focuses on providing an overview of advanced techniques in a practical, clinically useful fashion. Imaging, revision sinus surgery, frontal sinus surgery, postoperative care, and rhinoplasty are discussed. Endoscopic

0030-6665/06/$ - see front matter © 2006 Elsevier Inc. All rights reserved.
doi:10.1016/j.otc.2006.01.016

oto.theclinics.com

approaches to orbital surgery, such as endoscopic dacryocystorhinostomy and orbital and optic nerve decompression, are presented. The important technology of computer-aided surgery is described in detail. Current applications for lasers in rhinology are noted. Today, rhinologists are pursuing endoscopic approaches to the skull base, and thus, endoscopic techniques for transsphenoidal hypophysectomy and resection of fibro-osseous lesions, clivus tumors, and paranasal sinus neoplasms (benign and malignant) are explored.

Finally, we must acknowledge and thank the authors, whose contributions constitute the substance of this issue. This sharing of ideas in a public forum facilitates better patient care today. In addition, these efforts foster the creativity that will drive the future innovations that will help patients tomorrow.

Martin J. Citardi, MD, FACS
Pete S. Batra, MD
Section of Nasal and Sinus Disorders
The Cleveland Clinic Head and Neck Institute
9500 Euclid Avenue, Desk A71
Cleveland, OH 44195, USA

E-mail addresses: citardm@ccf.org,
batrap@ccf.org

ELSEVIER
SAUNDERS

Otolaryngol Clin N Am
39 (2006) 403–416

OTOLARYNGOLOGIC
CLINICS
OF NORTH AMERICA

Imaging for Functional Endoscopic Sinus Surgery

Nafi Aygun, MD[a],*, S. James Zinreich, MD[b]

[a]*Russell H. Morgan Department of Radiology and Radiological Sciences, The Johns Hopkins Medical Institution, 600 N. Wolfe Street/Phipps B-126-A, Baltimore, MD 21287, USA*
[b]*Russell H. Morgan Department of Radiology and Radiological Sciences, The Johns Hopkins Medical Institution, 600 N. Wolfe Street/Phipps B-100, Baltimore, MD 21287, USA*

Radiologic imaging is complementary to the clinical and endoscopic evaluation of patients with sinusitis, but not the primary way to diagnose this entity. The diagnosis of sinusitis is made clinically with the help of endoscopy. Imaging is an essential part of presurgical evaluation and of monitoring difficult-to-treat, recurrent, and postsurgical disease. In patients with noninflammatory sinus pathology and patients who "baffle" clinical diagnosis, imaging is extremely helpful in differentiating the various pathologic entities and determining the extent of disease.

Cross-sectional imaging has made plain films and plain film tomography obsolete. CT, when deemed clinically necessary, is the current modality of choice to evaluate sinusitis [1]. CT's ability to display bone, mucosa, and air makes it a perfect tool for imaging of the paranasal sinuses. The fine bony architecture of the nasal cavity and the paranasal sinus drainage pathways are depicted accurately with CT examination.

CT

Technique

Single channel CT (SC-CT) scanners use either incremental or helical acquisition schemes for paranasal sinus examinations. Image acquisition in the coronal plane is preferred for optimal display of the anterior ostiomeatal unit. The slice thickness should be 3 mm or less without interstice gap for optimal evaluation of key structures such as ostiomeatal unit and frontal recess. Image acquisition in the coronal plane requires extension of the head,

---

* Corresponding author.
E-mail address: Naygun1@jhmi.edu (N. Aygun).

0030-6665/06/$ - see front matter © 2006 Elsevier Inc. All rights reserved.
doi:10.1016/j.otc.2006.01.014
oto.theclinics.com

which may not be possible for some elderly patients and patients with air-way problems or neck pain. Thin axial images can be reconstructed in the coronal plane for such patients.

Multichannel CT (MC-CT) scanners (also called multidetector or multi-slice CT scanners) employ multiple rows of detectors that allow registration of multiple channels of data with one rotation of the radiograph tube. For example, a 16-slice MC-CT scanner has a 16-fold capacity for collecting image data per radiograph tube rotation, compared with an SC-CT. Currently, 64-channel CT scanners are in routine clinical use. A "head-to-toe" CT scan with slices as thin as 0.2 mm can be obtained in 60 seconds. Thin slices permit isotropic data sets, in which the voxels (the smallest elements of a data set) are cubical. Isotropic voxels afford excellent reconstruction of images in essentially any desired plane without degradation of image quality (Fig. 1). Isotropic imaging created a paradigm shift in CT imaging: one is no longer limited by the plane of acquisition. Data can be collected from a body part in any desired plane and two-dimensional images in any desired plane (multiplanar reconstruction or MPR) can be reconstructed. Real-time interactive manipulation of image data and three-dimensional reconstructions are made possible by high-performance workstations equipped with special software.

An innovative use of CT technology aimed at visualizing the ventilation processes of the nasal cavity and paranasal sinuses is xenon-CT [2–4]. Because of its radio-opaque property, xenon can be visualized with CT and allows quantitative evaluation of the ventilation rate. This technology is in its evolutionary phase and, it is hoped, will add significantly to the radiologic evaluation of the regional pathophysiology.

Flat-panel-based CT scanners will be introduced for routine clinical use in the very near future. These scanners have changed the image acquisition paradigm once again. Flat-panel-based CT, instead of building the volume from individual slices, acquires the image data volume directly. This provides seamless volume images, which undoubtedly will improve 2D and 3D reconstructions and model building capability for presurgical evaluation.

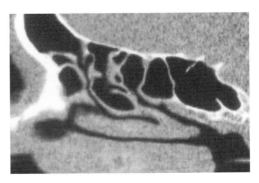

Fig. 1. Reconstructed sagittal CT image obtained from spiral CT data. As demonstrated by this image, these reconstructed images are equal in quality to the original data set obtained.

To what extent flat-panel-based CT will benefit radiologic imaging and intraoperative guidance is yet to be seen.

Radiation exposure

High-resolution imaging inevitably increases the radiation dose to patients. Factors inherent to the individual CT scanner and patient greatly influence the radiation dose [5–7]. Among the many operator-adjustable scanning parameters that affect the radiation dose, tube current (measured in milliamp-seconds or mA) has the most direct and profound effect on the final radiation dose received by the patient. A considerable reduction in radiation exposure can be achieved by lowering mA [8,9]. However, low mA result in increased image noise and possible loss of fine detail [9–12]. A tube current of 50 mA to 80 mA at 120 kilovolts peak (kVp) tube voltage is a reasonable compromise, and diagnostic accuracy of paranasal sinus CT is not affected at these settings compared with higher mA values [9–12]. The radiation exposure to the lens from sinus CT examination is well below the threshold level believed to induce cataracts; however, there is a theoretical risk of stochastic effects (eg, carcinogenesis), which is not dependent on a minimum threshold of exposure [13]. Therefore, judicious use of CT is advised. Specifically, multiple examinations with high-dose protocols should be avoided, especially in young patients and women of childbearing age.

MRI

The most significant advantage of MRI over CT is its exquisite contrast resolution, which allows differentiation of sinus secretions from mass lesions, brain, and orbital structures. Evaluation of neoplastic and invasive inflammatory processes of the paranasal sinuses is best accomplished by MRI. However, MRI often fails to evaluate the integrity of the thin bones of the anterior skull base. This limitation precludes the use of MRI in imaging inflammatory disease, despite its exquisite sensitivity in displaying mucosal changes.

T1- and T2-weighted MRI obtained in axial and coronal planes provide a satisfactory evaluation of the sinuses. Contrast-enhanced (gadolinium-diethylenetriamine pentaacetic acid [Gd-DTPA]), fat-saturated, T1-weighted images are indispensable for a more comprehensive examination, especially in patients with noninflammatory sinus pathology.

The high cost of MRI and its long image acquisition time continue to be problematic. Recent advances in coil technology and high field (3 Tesla or 3T) magnets provide faster imaging. However, paranasal sinus imaging does not benefit from this technology to the same degree as does brain imaging, due to the intimate presence of air and bone in this anatomic area, resulting in increased chemical shift and susceptibility artifacts at 3T.

Advanced imaging modalities

Advances in image acquisition technologies are paralleled by remarkable improvements in image display and image-guided surgery fields. New computer systems have been developed with software that fuses CT and MR images and reconstructs them into a three-dimensional image that can be incorporated into a stereotactic navigation system.

Image overlay is a visualization method that combines 3D computer-generated images with the user's view of the real world. Changes in the observer's viewpoint are tracked and computer images appear in appropriate locations, so the user sees virtual images registered within the real world scene. This provides a virtual "X-ray vision" to the surgeon, who can view the image data superimposed on the patient without looking away from the operative field. The concept of image overlay has the potential to radically change the surgeon's perception and reaction.

One of the most significant limitations of image-guided surgery systems is that the images are detained and reflect the preoperative morphology. Real-time intraoperative MRI is now a routine tool in many neurosurgical operating suites, but it is expensive and subject to the limitations associated with MR imaging. Real-time intraoperative CT is technically feasible but will require fundamental changes in operating room design and safety. Newer CT units are being developed that, although similar in capability to larger units, are much smaller in size, allowing them to be used in an office setting as well as the operating room.

Anatomy

We will briefly review the anatomy of the nasal cavity and paranasal sinuses by focusing on the three "tight spots": the frontal recess, the infundibular middle meatus, and the sphenoethmoid recess.

The frontal sinus drainage pathway is the most complex. This complexity, coupled with the common occurrence of anatomic variations, leads to a high number of failed surgeries. The bottom portion of the hourglass-shaped frontal sinus drainage pathway is called the frontal recess and is also the narrowest portion of this outflow tract. The frontal recess is neighbored by the agger nasi cell anteriorly, the ethmoid bulla posteriorly and the uncinate process inferiorly. The agger nasi cell is an ethmoturbinal remnant, which is present in almost all patients. It is aerated, and represents the most anterior ethmoid air cell. It usually borders the primary ostium, or floor, of the frontal sinus; thus, its size may directly influence the patency of the frontal recess and the anterior middle meatus. The uncinate process is a superior extension of the lateral nasal wall (the medial wall of the maxillary sinus). Anteriorly, the uncinate process fuses with the posteromedial wall of the agger nasi cell and the posteromedial wall of the nasolacrimal duct. Laterally, the free edge of the uncinate process delimits the infundibulum, which is the air passage that connects the maxillary sinus ostium to the middle meatus.

The superior attachment of the uncinate process has three major varia-tions that determine the anatomic configuration of the frontal recess and its drainage [14]. These variations are as follows.

- The uncinate process may extend laterally to attach to the lamina pap-yracea or the ethmoid bulla, forming a terminal recess of the infundib-ulum; the frontal recess opens directly to the middle meatus.
- The uncinate process may extend medially and attach to the lateral sur-face of the middle turbinate.
- The uncinate process may extend medially and superiorly to attach di-rectly to the skull base.

In the latter two forms, the frontal recess drains to the infundibulum.

The sphenoethmoidal recess receives drainage from the posterior ethmoid cells and the sphenoid sinus. It lies just lateral to the nasal septum and leads to the posterior aspect of the superior meatus. The sphenoethmoidal recess is vi-sualized on coronal images but is best evaluated in the sagittal and axial planes.

Using a coronal CT scan, one can visualize the anatomy of the frontal recess, infundibulum, and middle meatus. This is crucial for proper diagno-sis and treatment. Using the real-time multiplanar reconstruction capabil-ities of modern imaging work-stations, one can considerably advance his/her understanding of the complex anatomy of these regions. The authors found oblique coronal reconstructions with 20 degrees craniocaudal angula-tion and oblique sagittal reconstructions with 5 to 10 degrees lateromedial angulation to be particularly helpful in demonstrating the frontal-recess–agger-nasi-cell–uncinate-process relationship. Routine axial images show the sphenoethmoidal recess to our satisfaction but minimally obliqued sagittal reconstructions best demonstrate the sphenoethmoidal-recess–superior-meatus relationship.

Chronic rhinosinusitis

The most common indication for sinus imaging is chronic rhinosinusitis (CRS). CT is the imaging standard for evaluation of CRS [1]. The CT signs suggestive of CRS include diffuse or focal mucosal thickening, partial or complete opacification, bone remodeling and thickening caused by osteitis from adjacent chronic mucosal inflammation, and polyposis. The distribu-tion of the inflammatory mucosal changes in the nasal cavity and sinuses may provide a clue as to the level of mechanical obstruction that can be pin-pointed by evaluating the sinus drainage pathways. Although CT provides excellent information about the extent and distribution of mucosal disease and the status of the nasal air passages, it does not yield much information about the origin of the changes (eg, infection, allergies, granulomatous in-flammation, postsurgical scarring, and so forth).

When sinus secretions are acute and of low viscosity, they are of interme-diate attenuation on CT (10–25 Hounsfield units). In the more chronic state, sinus secretions become thickened and concentrated, and the CT attenuation increases, with density measurements of 30 to 60 Hounsfield units [15].

Sinonasal polyposis has been recognized as a distinct form of CRS both clinically and radiographically, although polyp formation is a nonspecific response to a variety of inflammatory stimuli. There is an obvious association with asthma, aspirin sensitivity, and eosinophilia.

Antrochoanal and sphenochoanal polyps appear as well-defined masses that arise from the maxillary or sphenoid sinus and extend to the choana through the middle meatus or sphenoethmoid recess, respectively. They can present as nasopharyngeal masses. It is important to recognize their origin and relationship to the maxillary or sphenoid ostium in treatment planning.

Retention cysts are common incidental findings on imaging studies and are seen as well-defined rounded masses, typically on the maxillary sinus floor. Their clinical significance is not clear [16]. They may become symptomatic if large enough to interfere with drainage pathways [17].

Mucocele, a complication of CRS, results from obstruction of the sinus drainage and subsequent expansion of the sinus. Mucoceles are seen more commonly in the ethmoid and frontal sinuses and present with symptoms secondary to compression of the adjacent structures, in addition to the usual symptoms of CRS.

Thickening and sclerosis of the bony walls of the sinuses are at least in part secondary to the spread of the inflammation through the haversian system within the bone [18,19].

On MRI, the appearance of CRS varies because of the changing concentrations of protein and free water protons (Fig. 2) [20]. Som and Curtin [15] describe four patterns of MRI signal intensity that can be seen with chronic sinusitis:

- Hypointense on T1-weighted images and hyperintense on T2-weighted images with a protein concentration of less than 9%
- Hyperintense on T1-weighted images and hyperintense on T2-weighted images with total protein concentration increased to 20%–25%
- Hyperintense on T1-weighted images and hypointense on T2-weighted images with total protein concentration of 25%–30%
- Hypointense on T1-weighted images and T2-weighted images with a protein concentration greater than 30% and inspissated secretions in an almost solid form

MRI of inspissated secretions (ie, those with protein concentrations greater than 30%) may have a pitfall in that the signal voids on T1- and T2-weighted images may look identical to normally aerated sinuses.

The correlation between patient symptoms and CT findings is difficult to determine partly because chronic mucosal inflammation may be present without CT findings and asymptomatic persons can have abnormal CT scans. Several studies failed to show a correlation between symptom severity

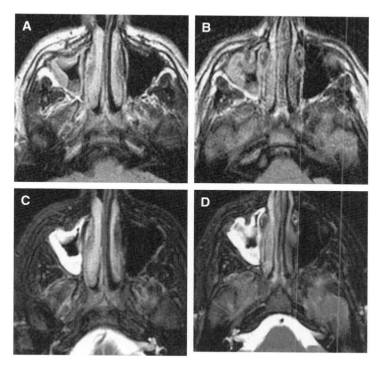

Fig. 2. T1-weighted images (*A, B*) and T2-weighted images (*C, D*). These images reveal the "classic" display of inflammatory disease within the right maxillary sinuses. The T2-weighted images optimally display the extent of inflammatory mucosa involvement of the sinuses.

and severity of CT findings [21–25]. In particular, symptoms such as headache and facial pain do not correlate with CT findings at all [26,27]. A positive correlation between the severity of symptoms and CT findings may be demonstrated when certain symptoms and negative CT exams are eliminated [28,29]. The nasal endoscopy findings correlate with CT findings, although the correlation is less than perfect [23,30,31]. The positive predictive value of abnormal endoscopy for abnormal CT is greater than 90%, whereas the negative predictive value of normal endoscopy for normal CT is only 70% [23,26].

To better classify patients into diagnostic and prognostic categories, various symptom, CT, and endoscopy scoring systems have been used. The Lund-MacKay scoring system is the most popular method used for CT description of sinus disease because of its simplicity and reproducibility [32]. A score of zero, one, or two is given to each of the five sites (anterior ethmoid, posterior ethmoid, frontal, maxillary and sphenoid) on both sides of the sinonasal cavity for normal pneumatization, partial opacification or complete opacification, respectively [33,34]. The ostiomeatal complex receives either zero or two. This yields a maximum score of 12 for one side. Unfortunately, the system is limited in levels of stratification (ie, the definition of partial opacification can range anywhere from 1% to 99%). Another limitation may be using inflammation as the basis of measurement, instead of the obstruction of the ostiomeatal channel, which may be more important. A classification system that provides evaluation of the ostiomeatal units and better stratification of mucosal disease is needed.

The impact of CT on treatment decision was evaluated in a small study [35]. CT changed the treatment in one third of the patients and allowed more agreement on treatment plan among ENT surgeons [35].

Fungal rhinosinusitis

The role of fungi in the development of CRS is an active area of research and it may not be prudent to discuss fungal rhinosinusitis (FRS) separately from CRS. Nonetheless, there are certain differences between CRS and FRS in patient demographics, diagnosis, treatment, and prognosis. Two main forms of FRS are differentiated: invasive and noninvasive [36]. Within these categories, five clinicopathologically distinct entities are defined [37]: acute invasive, chronic invasive granulomatous form, chronic invasive nongranulomatous form, fungus ball and allergic fungal sinusitis. It must be emphasized that FRS is a spectrum of disease and the differences in clinical presentation are largely determined by the host defense system. Therefore, it is not uncommon to see overlapping clinical and imaging features.

Acute invasive FRS is seen primarily in immunocompromised patients and is fatal if untreated, and often despite treatment. A high index of clinical suspicion and biopsy of the middle turbinate are necessary for early diagnosis, which may be life saving [38]. CT study obtained early in the disease course may be normal or show nonspecific mucosal thickening indistinguishable from the appearance of bacterial/viral disease [39]. Bone destruction and swelling of the soft tissues adjacent to the paranasal sinuses occur in advanced disease.

Chronic invasive FRS has been associated primarily with immunocompromised individuals; however, it does occur in the nonimmunocompromised. It has a more protracted course, with a relatively slow progression of disease, sometimes despite treatment, and a high recurrence rate. There is no apparent difference in clinical and radiologic features of the granulomatous and nongranulomatous forms. The radiologic hallmark of chronic invasive FRS is bone destruction, which is better depicted with CT, whereas MRI better defines the soft tissue extent of disease and brain involvement. Foci of increased attenuation (on CT) in the thickened sinus mucosa may indicate fungal colonization, as found in 74% of our patient population [40]. The radiologic differential diagnosis of chronic invasive FRS is broad and includes benign and malignant neoplasms, infectious and idiopathic granulomatous diseases, and allergic fungal sinusitis.

Fungus ball refers to a sinus mass that consists of packed hyphae. Patients with fungus ball are typically immunocompetent and they present with varying nonspecific sinus-related complaints. Serendipitous identification of fungus balls is not uncommon. Diffuse opacification of a single sinus is the most common radiographic feature [41]. Foci of hyperattenuation in the center of the sinus mass is seen in approximately 50% to 74% of patients [39,41,42]. Large calcified concretions are characteristic of the disease but found uncommonly. Thickening of the sinus walls is common. Bone erosion may be seen occasionally.

Allergic FRS, an immunologically mediated hypersensitivity reaction to fungi, is the most common fungal disease of the sinuses [43]. The authors suspect that there is a large overlap between CRS and allergic FRS. A central area of hyperattenuation on sinus CT is almost always present and corresponds to markedly decreased T2 signal on MRI. Examination of fungal concretions reveals the presence of iron and magnesium in quantities sufficient enough to affect the signal (Fig. 3) [40,44]. Others contend that the decreased signal is due to the dehydration of mucus [15]. Expansion of the involved sinuses with bone remodeling or destruction is common.

Saprophytic colonization of the sinonasal mucosa is very common, particularly in patients who have undergone sinus surgery, and the mere presence of fungi on the mucosa does not necessarily constitute disease.

Neoplasms of the sinonasal cavities

Squamous cell cancer arising from the sinonasal epithelium accounts for 80% of the malignant tumors seen in this body part. Adenocarcinomas arising from the minor salivary glands interspersed in the sinonasal mucosa account for up to 10% of the malignant tumors. Melanomas are responsible for 5% of sinonasal malignant tumors. Less common malignant tumors of the sinonasal cavities include olfactory neuroblastoma, lymphomas, and sarcomas. A detailed discussion of these individual entities is beyond the scope of this text. A list of commonly encountered tumors is provided in Box 1.

Diagnosis of malignant tumors is often delayed due to the low propensity of these tumors to elicit symptoms in the early stages. Symptoms are generally secondary to invasion of the skull base or orbit, perineural spread, and obstruction of a sinus ostium, and they occur later in the disease process. Some of the symptoms mimic inflammatory sinus disease and it is not uncommon for patients to be treated for rhinosinusitis before the diagnosis of malignancy is made. In the early stages of the disease, CT findings may be indistinguishable from those of inflammatory disease, which often accompanies neoplastic tissue. MR is better able to differentiate inflammatory disease from neoplasm but is not used routinely for the evaluation of inflammatory disease. The authors found that detection of erosion and destruction of the thin bones may allow one to diagnose these tumors while they are still

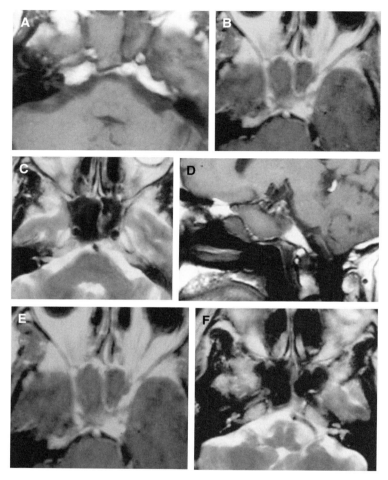

Fig. 3. MR of sphenoid fungal sinusitis. T1-weighted images (A, D), T1-weighted images post contrast (B, E), and T2- weighted images (C, F) reveal the lack of signal intensity within the fungal concretion on the T-2weighted images. Note the difference between these findings and those associated with bacterial/viral inflammatory disease.

in the sinonasal cavity, which requires careful examination of all sinus CT findings with the possibility of a malignancy in mind.

Appropriate treatment of sinonasal tumors requires an accurate preoperative depiction of tumor extent. Knowledge of the pathways of disease spread is important when interpreting these images. In general, CT is more accurate for the evaluation of bone integrity, whereas MRI is superior to CT in assessing the extent of disease and in differentiating the tumor from secondary inflammatory changes. In our practice, most patients are imaged with both MRI and CT before surgery.

Box 1. Common neoplasms of the sinonasal cavities

Epthelial
Epidermoid
   Squamous cell carcinoma
   Papilloma
Nonepidermoid
   Adeno carcinoma
   Adenoid cystic carcinoma
   Mucoepidermoid carcinoma
   Acinic cell carcinoma
   Adenoma
   Oncocytoma
Neuroectodermal
   Olfactory neuroblastoma
   Melanoma
Lymphomas
Sarcomas
Metastases
Osseous
   Osteoma
   Osteoblastoma
   Giant cell tumor
   Fibrous dysplasia
   Ossifying dysplasia
Odontogenic
   Ameloblastoma
   Calcifying epithelial odontogenic tumor
Vascular
   Hemangioma
   Juvenile angiofibroma

There are two very important questions to answer in preoperative evaluation:

1. Is the periorbita breeched?
2. Is the dura invaded?

Most surgeons believe that periorbital invasion requires orbital exenteration. Preoperative determination of invasion of the periorbita is difficult because a tumor can destruct the bone and indent on the periorbita without breeching it. Therefore, bone destruction does not necessitate periorbital invasion. Similarly, a tumor apparently bulging into the orbit may be confined by the intact periorbita. Infiltration or stranding of the periorbital fat tissue and nodularity of the interface between the tumor and orbital tissue are more reliable signs of periorbital invasion [45]. The authors have found high resolution fat-saturated T1-weighted images to be particularly helpful in this scenario. The overall accuracy of imaging for determination of presence or absence of periorbital invasion is about 60% to 70% [45]. It is important to note that this modest accuracy is mainly a reflection of a low negative predictive value. Thus, the presence of periorbital invasion is predicted more accurately than the absence of invasion.

Intracranial extension of tumor and invasion of the dura are important to identify because of their impact on treatment and prognosis. MRI is the modality of choice in this scenario. When there is irregular/nodular thickening and enhancement of the dura or smooth thickening of the dura of more than 5 mm, the diagnosis of dural invasion can be made with a 100% positive predictive value [46]. Difficulty arises when the thickening and enhancement are smooth and thin, which can be seen both with dural invasion and reactive changes. As in the periorbital invasion, it is easier to confirm the presence of invasion than the absence of it.

Perineural spread is another way by which sinonasal tumors can invade intracranial structures. Imaging can demonstrate perineural spread of disease before the patient becomes symptomatic, dramatically changing the course of treatment. Detection of perineural metastasis requires detailed knowledge of skull base anatomy and good-quality images. MRI is far superior to CT in this respect. High resolution fat-suppressed T1-weighted images are extremely helpful for this diagnosis. The evaluation of the pterygopalatine fossa (PPF) is particularly important because in the majority of cases the tumor first involves the PPF before it infiltrates the inferior orbital fissure, foramen rotundum, foramen ovale, vidian canal, and finally cavernous sinus and Meckel's cave.

Positron emission tomography (PET) is a very robust tool in oncological imaging in general. Unfortunately, PET and PET-CT have important shortcomings in the evaluation of skull base and sinonasal tumors. Lower resolution than that of CT and MRI is a major disadvantage in this anatomic area where the normal, as well as abnormal, structures of interest are often very small. PET does not perform as well as MRI in T staging of untreated patients. However, for the detection of distant metastases, PET has a clear advantage over the other modalities. Similarly, PET can provide information that is otherwise unavailable in the evaluation of patients after surgery and radiotherapy.

References

[1] Benninger MS, Ferguson BJ, Hadley JA, et al. Adult chronic rhinosinusitis: definitions, diagnosis, epidemiology, and pathophysiology. Otolaryngol Head Neck Surg 2003;129:S1–32.

[2] Paulsson B, Lindberg S, Ohlin P. Washout of 133-xenon as an objective assessment of para-nasal sinus ventilation in endoscopic sinus surgery. Ann Otol Rhinol Laryngol 2002;111: 710–7.

[3] Brumund KT, Graham SM, Beck KC, et al. The effect of maxillary sinus antrostomy size on xenon ventilation in the sheep model. Otolaryngol Head Neck Surg 2004;131:528–33.

[4] Marcucci C, Leopold DA, Cullen M, et al. Dynamic assessment of paranasal sinus ventila-tion using xenon-enhanced computed tomography. Ann Otol Rhinol Laryngol 2001;110: 968–75.

[5] Dammann F, Momino-Traserra E, Remy C, et al. Strahlenexposition bei der spiral-CT der nasennebenhöhlen. [Radiation exposure during spiral-CT of the paranasal sinuses]. ROFO 2000;172:232–7.

[6] Duvoisin B, Landry M, Chapuis L, et al. Low-dose CT and inflammatory disease of the para-nasal sinuses. Neuroradiology 1991;33:403–6.

[7] Hagtvedt T, Aalokken TM, Notthellen J, et al. A new low-dose CT examination compared with standard-dose CT in the diagnosis of acute sinusitis. Eur Radiol 2003;13:976–80.

[8] Hein E, Rogalla P, Klingebiel R, et al. Low-dose CT of the paranasal sinuses with eye lens protection: effect on image quality and radiation dose. Eur Radiol 2002;12:1693–6.

[9] Sohaib SA, Peppercorn PD, Horrocks JA, et al. The effect of decreasing mAs on image qual-ity and patient dose in sinus CT. Br J Radiol 2001;74:157–61.

[10] Kearney SE, Jones P, Meakin K, et al. CT scanning of the paranasal sinuses–the effect of reducing mAs. Br J Radiol 1997;70:1071–4.

[11] Tack D, Widelec J, De Maertelaer V, et al. Comparison between low-dose and standard-dose multidetector CT in patients with suspected chronic sinusitis. AJR Am J Roentgenol 2003; 181:939–44.

[12] Zammit-Maempel I, Chadwick CL, Willis SP. Radiation dose to the lens of eye and thyroid gland in paranasal sinus multislice CT. Br J Radiol 2003;76:418–20.

[13] Czechowski J, Janeczek J, Kelly G, et al. Radiation dose to the lens in sequential and spiral CT of the facial bones and sinuses. Eur Radiol 2001;11:711–3.

[14] Daniels DL, Mafee MF, Smith MM, et al. The frontal sinus drainage pathway and related structures. AJNR Am J Neuroradiol 2003;24:1618–27.

[15] Som PM, Curtin HD. Chronic inflammatory sinonasal diseases including fungal infections. The role of imaging. Radiol Clin North Am 1993;31:33–44.

[16] Bhattacharyya N. Do maxillary sinus retention cysts reflect obstructive sinus phenomena? Arch Otolaryngol Head Neck Surg 2000;126:1369–71.

[17] Hadar T, Shvero J, Nageris BI, et al. Mucus retention cyst of the maxillary sinus: the endo-scopic approach. Br J Oral Maxillofac Surg 2000;38:227–9.

[18] Perloff JR, Gannon FH, Bolger WE, et al. Bone involvement in sinusitis: an apparent path-way for the spread of disease. Laryngoscope 2000;110:2095–9.

[19] Khalid AN, Hunt J, Perloff JR, et al. The role of bone in chronic rhinosinusitis. Laryngo-scope 2002;112:1951–7.

[20] Som PM, Dillon WP, Fullerton GD, et al. Chronically obstructed sinonasal secretions: observations on T1 and T2 shortening. Radiology 1989;172:515–20.

[21] Bhattacharyya T, Piccirillo J, Wippold FJ II. Relationship between patient-based descrip-tions of sinusitis and paranasal sinus computed tomographic findings. Arch Otolaryngol Head Neck Surg 1997;123:1189–92.

[22] Stankiewicz JA, Chow JM. A diagnostic dilemma for chronic rhinosinusitis: definition accu-racy and validity. Am J Rhinol 2002;16:199–202.

[23] Stankiewicz JA, Chow JM. Nasal endoscopy and the definition and diagnosis of chronic rhinosinusitis. Otolaryngol Head Neck Surg 2002;126:623–7.

[24] Stewart MG, Sicard MW, Piccirillo JF, et al. Severity staging in chronic sinusitis: are CT scan findings related to patient symptoms? Am J Rhinol 1999;13:161–7.

[25] Ashraf N, Bhattacharyya N. Determination of the "incidental" Lund score for the staging of chronic rhinosinusitis. Otolaryngol Head Neck Surg 2001;125:483–6.

[26] Rosbe KW, Jones KR. Usefulness of patient symptoms and nasal endoscopy in the diagnosis of chronic sinusitis. Am J Rhinol 1998;12:167–71.

[27] Mudgil SP, Wise SW, Hopper KD, et al. Correlation between presumed sinusitis-induced pain and paranasal sinus computed tomographic findings. Ann Allergy Asthma Immunol 2002;88:223–6.

[28] Kenny TJ, Duncavage J, Bracikowski J, et al. Prospective analysis of sinus symptoms and correlation with paranasal computed tomography scan. Otolaryngol Head Neck Surg 2001;125:40–3.

[29] Arango P, Kountakis SE. Significance of computed tomography pathology in chronic rhinosinusitis. Laryngoscope 2001;111:1779–82.

[30] Rose GE, Sandy C, Hallberg L, et al. Clinical and radiologic characteristics of the imploding antrum, or "silent sinus," syndrome. Ophthalmology 2003;110:811–8.

[31] Kennedy DW, Wright ED, Goldberg AN. Objective and subjective outcomes in surgery for chronic sinusitis. Laryngoscope 2000;110:29–31.

[32] Friedman WH, Katsantonis GP. Staging systems for chronic sinus disease. Ear Nose Throat J 1994;73:480–4.

[33] Lund VJ, Kennedy DW. Quantification for staging sinusitis. The staging and therapy group. Ann Otol Rhinol Laryngol Suppl 1995;167:17–21.

[34] Lund VJ, Mackay IS. Staging in rhinosinusitus. Rhinology 1993;31:183–4.

[35] Anzai Y, Yueh B. Imaging evaluation of sinusitis: diagnostic performance and impact on health outcome. Neuroimaging Clin N Am 2003;13:251–63 [xi.].

[36] deShazo RD, O'Brien M, Chapin K, et al. A new classification and diagnostic criteria for invasive fungal sinusitis. Arch Otolaryngol Head Neck Surg 1997;123:1181–8.

[37] Ferguson BJ. Definitions of fungal rhinosinusitis. Otolaryngol Clin North Am 2000;33: 227–35.

[38] Gillespie MB, Huchton DM, O'Malley BW. Role of middle turbinate biopsy in the diagnosis of fulminant invasive fungal rhinosinusitis. Laryngoscope 2000;110:1832–6.

[39] DelGaudio JM, Swain RE Jr, Kingdom TT, et al. Computed tomographic findings in patients with invasive fungal sinusitis. Arch Otolaryngol Head Neck Surg 2003;129:236–40.

[40] Zinreich SJ, Kennedy DW, Malat J, et al. Fungal sinusitis: diagnosis with CT and MR imaging. Radiology 1988;169:439–44.

[41] Klossek JM, Serrano E, Peloquin L, et al. Functional endoscopic sinus surgery and 109 mycetomas of paranasal sinuses. Laryngoscope 1997;107:112–7.

[42] Dhong HJ, Jung JY, Park JH. Diagnostic accuracy in sinus fungus balls: CT scan and operative findings. Am J Rhinol 2000;14:227–31.

[43] Manning SC, Holman M. Further evidence for allergic pathophysiology in allergic fungal sinusitis. Laryngoscope 1998;108:1485–96.

[44] Zinreich SJ, Mattox DE, Kennedy DW, et al. Concha bullosa: CT evaluation. J Comput Assist Tomogr 1988;12:778–84.

[45] Eisen MD, Yousem DM, Loevner LA, et al. Preoperative imaging to predict orbital invasion by tumor. Head Neck 2000;22:456–62.

[46] Eisen MD, Yousem DM, Montone KT, et al. Use of preoperative MR to predict dural, perineural, and venous sinus invasion of skull base tumors. AJNR Am J Neuroradiol 1996;17: 1937–45.

ELSEVIER
SAUNDERS

Otolaryngol Clin N Am
39 (2006) 417–435

OTOLARYNGOLOGIC
CLINICS
OF NORTH AMERICA

Revision Endoscopic Sinus Surgery

Noam A. Cohen, MD, PhD, David W. Kennedy, MD*

Division of Rhinology, Department of Otorhinolaryngology–Head and Neck Surgery,
University of Pennsylvania School of Medicine, 5th floor Ravdin Building,
Hospital of the University of Pennsylvania, 3400 Spruce Street, Philadelphia, PA 19104

Functional endoscopic sinus surgery (FESS) has a long-term high rate of success (approximately 90%) for symptomatic improvement in patients with medically refractory chronic rhinosinusitis [1]. As the popularity of the technique continues to grow, however, so does the population of patients with postsurgical persistent sinus disease. This subset of patients often represents a challenge to the otorhinolaryngologist. Essential to management of these patients is identification of the source of persistent disease. These etiologies are best classified broadly as environmental, host, or iatrogenic. Although the focus of this article is iatrogenic issues, the topic of revision FESS cannot be discussed fully without mentioning environmental or host factors.

The central dogma of FESS is restoration of the natural sinus physiology (ie, mucociliary clearance). Environmental factors that pose a risk to the mucociliary apparatus, through toxicity or induction of mucosal inflammation, must be minimized if not outright eliminated. Common factors include air pollutants, allergens, tobacco smoke, and mold. Likewise, host factors that hinder mucociliary clearance or result in excessive inflammation must be reversed or improved. Questions addressing systemic disease, such as asthma, aspirin intolerance, immunodeficiencies, cystic fibrosis, granulomatous disease, primary ciliary dyskinesia, and neoplasia, should be asked. Nasal polyposis is a common cause for revision surgery and is most likely a manifestation of a combination of environmental exposure with excessive host response. Even with a well-executed surgical dissection, in the absence of addressing environmental and host mucociliary risk factors, failure is imminent in primary and revision surgery.

Iatrogenic disease may result from poor surgical technique, inadequate postoperative cavity débridement, or inadequate postoperative medical care. Mucosal preservation is paramount for success. Surgical technique

* Corresponding author.
E-mail address: david.kennedy@uphs.upenn.edu (D.W. Kennedy).

0030-6665/06/$ - see front matter © 2006 Elsevier Inc. All rights reserved.
doi:10.1016/j.otc.2006.01.003

that does not incorporate through-cutting forceps and directed powered mucosal shaving is prone to strip excessive mucosa resulting in underlying bony exposure and subsequent osteoneogenesis or osteitis (Fig. 1). Inflammation within the bone not only is difficult to eradicate, but also is likely to act as a nidus for local production of inflammatory mediators resulting in surrounding persistent mucosal disease and inhibition of mucosal healing [2–4]. Circumferential mucosal resection, especially at sinus ostia, predisposes the ostia to circumferential scarring during the healing process. Mucosal stripping may result in excessive scarring, which can cause lateralization of the middle turbinate or synechiae formation (Fig. 2). Inappropriately placed surgical ostia that do not encompass or communicate with the natural ostia generate a recirculation phenomenon, whereby mucus is swept by the mucosal apparatus out the natural ostium, only to reenter the sinus through the surgical antrostomy (Fig. 3) [5]. This recirculation loop is prone to contamination and persistent infection. Lastly, incomplete dissection often occurs in the ethmoid cavity, resulting in retained ethmoid partitions that act as a common source for persistent skull base and frontal recess polypoid degeneration.

Diagnosis

Identification of the cause of persistent postsurgical sinus disease requires a thorough history, nasal endoscopy, and a recent CT scan obtained after maximal medical therapy [6,7]. The initial step in the evaluation of a patient with persistent symptoms is consideration of the indications for the initial surgical procedure. After a prior surgery, the presence of scarring or the presence of some mucosal inflammation, even when this was not present before the prior surgery, can fool a surgeon seeing the patient for the first time

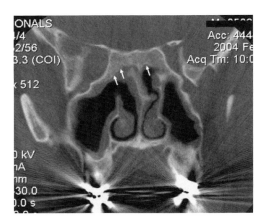

Fig. 1. CT scan of a patient who had undergone several previous sinus surgeries showing massively osteitic and thickened bone of the skull base (*arrows*) and bony septum.

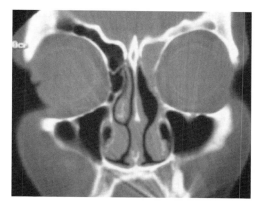

Fig. 2. CT scan showing a lateralized left middle turbinate adherent to the medial orbital wall. Improper identification of this postsurgical alteration could lead to dissection medially into the olfactory cleft resulting in violation of the cribriform plate.

into thinking that these changes are the cause of the patient's symptoms. Accordingly, whenever possible, the revision surgeon should obtain original records and radiographs for review. Occasionally, patients are identified whose initial CT scan shows minimal or no evidence of chronic

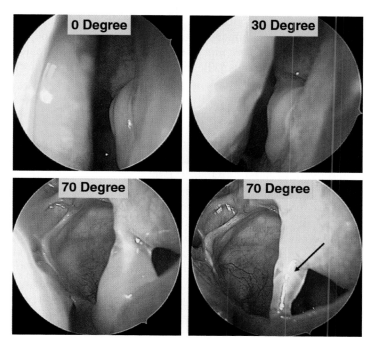

Fig. 3. Endoscopy of mucus from the maxillary sinus. Careful inspection with angled endoscopes shows mucus recirculation, which is confirmed by suctioning the mucus and revealing a bridge of tissue (arrow).

inflammation, and the indication for surgical intervention was headache or facial pain. In such situations, the recent presenting complaint must be interrogated thoroughly, and the surgeon must be convinced that it is of rhinologic origin because it is incumbent on the surgeon not to operate a second time for nonrhinologic complaints.

After evaluation of the indications for the primary surgery, the surgical technique and the prior postoperative period should be evaluated: Was the surgery a mucosal-preserving operation, were appropriate antibiotics and anti-inflammatories used, and was an adequate schedule of attentive postoperative débridement completed? Careful evaluation of the immediate 3-month postoperative period may give clues to some of the underlying causes of disease recurrence. Patients presenting for revision FESS typically are frustrated with the medical establishment and often turn to alternative medical therapies. The effects of alternative medical therapies are not well understood, and the use of these alternative therapies may complicate subsequent surgical intervention.

Nasal saline irrigation is often used as a helpful adjunct in the treatment of recurrent sinusitis patients [8]. Irrigation is fraught with potential difficulties, however. The source of the saline, the method of administration, and the sources of possible cross-contamination should be investigated. In cases in which the solution is not sterile or is prepared with water that might be contaminated, there is a concern for reinoculation of bacteria, especially *Pseudomonas* [9]. It is recommended to use sterile bottled saline or at least boiled or distilled water, keeping the solution refrigerated to lessen the chance of contamination, and at the same time to ensure adequate cleansing of the delivery device.

Nasal endoscopy

Nasal endoscopy is a crucial part of the evaluation of patients with chronic rhinosinusitis. The importance of nasal endoscopy cannot be emphasized enough, especially in patients with recurrent disease after surgical intervention. Most surgically created mechanical problems can be identified by nasal endoscopy, and some may be addressed and corrected in the outpatient clinic with topical or local infiltration of anesthetic.

A lateralized scarred middle turbinate with secondary obstruction is a common cause of failure after endoscopic sinus surgery. With attention to mucosal preservation technique, performing a controlled septal-turbinate synechiae (Bolgerization) at the end of the procedure [10], placing middle meatal sponges, and performing postoperative débridements, the likelihood of this outcome can be minimized.

Endoscopic visualization also can allow diagnosis of a missed ostium of the maxillary sinus. To ensure that the natural ostium was included in the maxillary antrostomy with no anterior scarring, a 45° or 70° angled telescope is often necessary (Fig. 3). The angled telescope also can visualize disease in a residual infraorbital (Haller) cell. In persistent maxillary sinus disease, it is important to evaluate the frontal recess. Persistent disease and drainage from the frontal area into the maxillary sinus may cause persistent maxillary sinusitis. Postsurgical endoscopic findings common for persistent sphenoid disease include circumferential scarring of the ostium and scarred superior turbinate, whereas findings consistent with persistent frontal sinus disease include a retained superior uncinate process, disease in an agar nasi cell, lateralized middle turbinate remnant, and bony spicules embedded in the mucosa resulting in persistent polypoid degeneration in the narrowest portion of the frontal recess (Fig. 4).

Radiology

A crucial aspect of the evaluation of postsurgical persistent disease is scrutiny of the postoperative CT scan. The middle meatal antrostomy should be examined for aspects of retained uncinate process in the region of the natural ostium of the maxillary sinus or unventilated cells missed on the primary procedure, such as the infraorbital (Haller) cells (Fig. 5). The frontal recesses should be identified, and patency should be determined. Postoperative recurrent frontal disease often is caused by persistent obstruction of the recess secondary to an undissected frontal cell, supraorbital ethmoid cell, or an agger nasi cell, any one of which would narrow the frontal recess (Fig. 6). Incomplete dissection of the posterior ethmoid cavity or scarring of the face of the sphenoid causes obstruction of the sphenoid without ever addressing the sphenoid surgically. Careful attention should be paid to the underlying bone for evidence of osteitis represented radiographically as thickened irregular bone (Fig. 7; see Figs. 1 and 5). Often axial images through the floor of the frontal sinus and frontal recess and through the sphenoid greatly aid in identifying the drainage pathway and often pinpoint the site of frontal sinus or sphenoid obstruction.

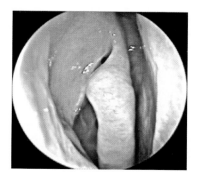

Fig. 4. Endoscopic appearance of incomplete uncinectomy, which often leads to persistent frontal recess disease.

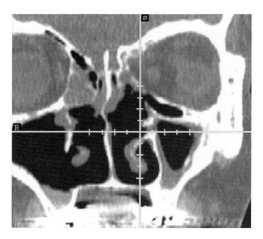

Fig. 5. Postsurgical CT scan showing a partially resected left infraorbital (Haller) cell with some thickened bone attached to it (possibly residual uncinate) There is persistent maxillary mucosal thickening.

The advent of interactive computer-assisted frameless stereotactic surgical navigation (stereotactic navigation) has revolutionized revision surgery. With the aid of stereotactic navigation, many high-risk areas have become easier to access safely endoscopically. Even more important, the ability to scroll through the radiographic anatomy in three dimensions simultaneously in advance of any surgical procedure allows for thorough conceptualization

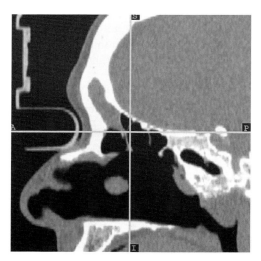

Fig. 6. Sagittal reconstruction CT scan showing unresected superior aspect, "the cap" of the agger nasi cell resulting in a narrowed frontal recess and frontal sinusitis. There is marked neo-osteogenesis in the region of the sphenoid sinus.

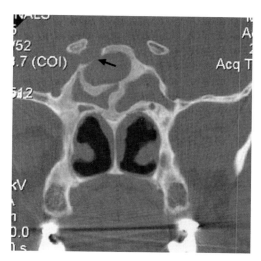

Fig. 7. Coronal CT scan showing thickened osteitic sphenoid bone with a bony dehiscence (*arrow*) adjacent to the right carotid.

of the altered three-dimensional anatomy and frequently helps to identify sources of obstruction and possible anatomic factors in persistent sinus disease.

Although not yet a standard of care, the American Academy of Otolaryngology–Head and Neck Surgery supports the use of stereotactic navigational surgery for the following clinical scenarios (http://www.entlink.net/practice/rules/image-guiding.cfm):

1. Revision sinus surgery
2. Distorted sinus anatomy of development, postoperative, or traumatic origins
3. Extensive sinonasal polyposis
4. Pathology involving the frontal, posterior ethmoid, and sphenoid sinuses
5. Disease abutting the skull base, orbit, optic nerve, or carotid artery
6. Cerebrospinal fluid (CSF) rhinorrhea or conditions in which there is a skull base defect
7. Benign and malignant sinonasal neoplasms

Stereotactic navigation has been shown to be beneficial in revision frontal sinus surgery [11] and may help reduce the rate of major complications [12]. Traditional frontal sinus procedures, such as osteoplastic flap with obliteration and external ethmoidectomy, have largely been replaced by endoscopic techniques, which significantly decrease patient morbidity and cosmetic deformity. Technologic breakthroughs, including stereotactic navigation systems such as intraoperative nerve monitoring, are no substitute for sound surgical anatomic knowledge. The major danger of using this technology is overreliance. The technology is still susceptible to displacement of the registration hardware and computer malfunction, and repeated visual confirmation of registration should be performed during surgery [13].

Although CT is the primary diagnostic modality for sinus disease, MRI is adjunctive and almost mandated in certain situations. MRI is particularly important when CT reveals opacification adjacent to a dehiscent skull base. In this situation, MRI identifies whether the erosion is secondary to sinus disease or secondary to a prior skull base erosion or trauma with resultant meningoencephalocele. The evaluation of dehiscent areas becomes even more crucial when located in the sphenoid adjacent to the carotid artery (Fig. 7). Iatrogenic injury to this region easily can result in formation of a carotid artery aneurysm or pseudoaneurysm. Additionally, it has been reported that fungal infections within the sphenoid can result in carotid involvement [14]. In these situations, magnetic resonance angiography also is employed, and the surgeon should consider angiography for even more detail.

MRI also enables differentiation of sinus and intranasal soft tissue masses. The thick dehydrated mucus of allergic fungal sinus or a fungus ball shows decreased resonance on the T_2-weighted images. A mucocele has varying densities based on water content, but usually is bright on T_1-weighted and T_2-weighted images. Another important role for MRI is in a tumor patient, in whom it enables differentiation of tumor from retained secretions. MRI also may help in radiologic differentiation of inverted papilloma from other tumors. Inverted papilloma typically shows "palisading" on MRI, whereas this pattern of resonance is unusual with other tumors.

Several studies investigating the cause of postsurgical recurrent sinusitis have been performed. Chu et al [15], reporting on 153 patients requiring revision endoscopic sinus surgery, found the most common surgical alteration associated with recurrent sinus disease was partial middle turbinectomy resulting in middle meatal scarring and lateralization of the middle turbinate. Ramadan [16] evaluated 52 cases of postsurgical persistent disease and reported that the most common cause of failure was residual air cells and adhesions in the ethmoid area (30.7%), followed by maxillary sinus ostial stenosis (27%), frontal sinus ostial stenosis (25%), and a separate maxillary sinus ostium stenosis in 15% of the cases. Musy and Kountakis [17], reporting on 70 patients, found that the most common postsurgical finding associated with primary surgery failure was lateralization of the middle turbinate (78%), followed by incomplete anterior ethmoidectomy (64%), scarred frontal recess (50%), incomplete posterior ethmoidectomy (41%), and middle meatal antrostomy stenosis (39%). These investigators reported a retained agger nasi cell and retained uncinate process in 49% and 37% of the patients; recurrent polyposis was identified in 37% of the patients [17]. Chiu and Vaughn [11], addressing revision frontal sinus surgery in 67 patients, found residual agger nasi cell or ethmoid bulla remnants in 79.1% of cases, remnant of superior uncinate process in 38.8%, lateralized middle turbinate remnant in 35.8%, polyps or polypoid mucosa in 29.9%, unopened frontal recess cells in 11.9%, and neo-osteogenesis of frontal recess in 4.5%. Although it is tempting in reviewing these reports to begin to think that the primary cause of failure to resolve disease is residual bony partitions or scarring, probably more often than not, the cause may be significantly due to nonsurgical factors, such as environmental allergies, mold exposure, hyperreactive mucosa, or other host factors affecting mucociliary clearance or propensity to infection.

Preoperative management

After the correct diagnosis is established, appropriate medical management is in place, and the disease is determined likely to be benefited by further surgery, multiple steps can be performed to optimize outcomes. Purulent secretions should be cultured, and appropriate culture-directed antibiotics should be administered in a patient with prior sinus surgery. The existence of nasal polyps or hyperplastic polypoid mucosa signals an increased risk of bleeding. Medical preparation of the surgical bed with oral steroids helps to stabilize the mucosa and to reduce bleeding during surgical intervention. If there are no contraindications to their use, preoperative steroids, 20 to 40 mg/d for 4 to 10 days, reduce polyp size and stabilize the inflammatory element found in the mucosa. In the preoperative setting, appropriate expectations should be set. Additionally, emphasis must be placed on the postoperative treatment plan, including medications and intensive endoscopic-guided débridements. With the exception of situations with imminent grave complications (encephaloceles, expansile mucoceles with bony remodeling), revision surgical intervention should not be performed in patients who are not willing to commit to aggressive postsurgical care.

Revision sinus surgery

Revision endoscopic sinus surgery is often substantially more complex than primary surgery because essential landmarks, such as the middle turbinate, uncinate process, basal lamella, and lamina papyracea, frequently may have been removed or drastically altered. The skull base, lamina papyracea, and other natural barriers to complications may have been eroded or entered at the prior surgical procedure. Lastly, patients requiring revision surgery often have massive nasal polyposis. It is imperative during surgery to identify the existing remaining surgical landmarks.

As noted earlier, the most common anatomic alteration from prior surgery is partial or total amputation of the middle turbinate. If the revision surgeon fails to recognize the remnant of middle turbinate, the ensuing dissection proceeds medially into the olfactory cleft or into the superior-posterior portion of the ethmoid cavity. Frequently, resection of the anterior portion of the middle turbinate gives rise to a small "uniturbinate," consisting of the fused superior remnant of the middle turbinate and the superior turbinate. In some cases, the superior attachment of the inferior turbinate, the posterior attachment of the middle turbinate, and the superior turbinate may be the only turbinate landmarks left [18]. The turbinate should be used with caution in a revision surgical procedure. Additionally, in severe polyposis, the residual middle turbinate may be pushed laterally by polyp growth medial to it; failure to recognize this before surgery may lead the surgeon into the rima olfactoria and increase the risk of intracranial entry. It is important that the primary landmarks in revision surgery remain the roof of the maxillary sinus, the medial orbital wall, and the skull base, and these landmarks should be identified carefully.

Surgical steps

As with all surgical procedures, but especially in revision surgery, the surgeon needs to work from "known" to "unknown." When the middle turbinate is medialized, and the uncinate is removed in its entirety, the maxillary sinus should be addressed. The posterior and superior walls of the sinus can be used as landmarks for further surgery. The medial orbital wall is identified and provides the next critical landmark. Failure to identify the medial orbital wall early may lead to dissection in the medial part of the ethmoid cavity, where the skull base is thin and downsloping, at a point in the surgery where adequate visualization of the anatomy has not been achieved.

Revision surgery techniques

General

It is paramount to have hard copies of the most recent radiographic studies hanging in the operating room. During the surgical procedure, these films should be reviewed multiple times. Although stated several times, it cannot be emphasized enough: Every time a sinus is approached, the radiographic anatomy should be studied, conceptualized, and endoscopically confirmed.

Before initiating surgery, adequate decongestion and vasoconstriction is necessary to minimize bleeding and maximize visualization. This is accomplished with topical vasoconstriction with oxymetazoline or cocaine and the injection of 1% xylocaine with 1:100,000 or 1:200,000 epinephrine. If posterior surgery is planned, injection of the sphenopalatine neurovascular bundle with lidocaine with 1:100,000 epinephrine greatly helps to decrease bleeding. This injection may be accomplished transnasally or transorally if the nasal cavity is obstructed with polyps. Transnasal injection is performed using an angled tonsil needle, which perforates the horizontal ground lamella in a lateral and upward direction. The foramen is palpated with the tip of the needle, and 1.5 mL of solution is injected slowly. Transoral injection is performed using a 25-gauge, 1.5-inch needle on a 3-mL syringe. The needle is bent 90°, 2.5 cm from the tip. The foramen can be palpated as a dimple in the palate medial to the second molar. The needle is inserted through the mucosa, and the foramen is identified by moving the tip of the needle along the palatine bone. When the canal is entered, the needle is inserted until the bend. The syringe is aspirated for blood to ensure not being intravascular. The injection is performed slowly taking care to aspirate several times during the injection with a total of 1.5 mL being injected. A blanching of the hemipalate is often an indication of a good injection. Temporary diplopia and visual loss have been noted with sphenopalatine injections.

When lateralizing the middle turbinate in a revision case, it is wise to review the extent of neo-osteogenesis in the turbinate before attempting to move it. In some cases, the middle turbinate can become significantly thicker than the adjacent skull base, creating the potential for skull base fracture and CSF leak. Synechiae should be taken down with a sharp sickle knife or through cutting forceps.

Osteitic bone often is encountered during revision surgery. To minimize postoperative inflammation and accelerate the healing, this bone should be débrided. Curets and grasping pistol grip forceps, such as a 45° upbiting Blakesley, are used with a "light" touch to remove osteitic bone. In instances of profuse thickened osteitic bone, a suction irrigation drill may be necessary to remove the diseased bone. The 70° suction irrigation drill is extremely helpful for removing bone from the region of the frontal recess.

Maxillary sinus

Persistent maxillary sinus disease, as in other persistent disease, may be a reflection of a general host or environmental cause of persistent rhinosinusitis. The common local problems that are encountered with a diseased maxillary sinus can be clustered into five large categories: recirculation, infection draining into the maxillary sinus from elsewhere, retained foreign body (including infected dental work), failure of mucociliary transport, and scar separation of the sinus from the nasal cavity [5,19]. Additionally, the possibility of local osteitis should be considered.

The recirculation phenomenon described previously may be caused by a retained or partially resected uncinate process with an iatrogenic posterior fontanelle antrostomy or, less frequently, by scarring at the anterior aspect of the antrostomy. The treatment at surgery is to resect the intervening tissue—this removes the bridge generating the recirculation. A 45° or 70° scope is required to see these regions and to ensure that residual uncinate or scarring is not present within this region. A technique for dissection and removal of residual uncinate involves use of the backbiter. Insertion of the backbiter into the maxillary sinus with gentle traction anteriorly lodges the crotch of the instrument on the anterior-most portion of the antrostomy. The instrument is partially closed, and a gentle rotation superiorly (counterclockwise—left; clockwise—right) is performed. This motion pulls the retained uncinate medially away from anterior and superior scar tissue. The uncinate is grasped with a forceps and removed. To avoid injury to the nasolacrimal duct, care must be taken not to force the instrument anteriorly.

A diseased residual infraorbital cell (Haller), even when opened, may have residual osteitic partitions, creating persistent localized mucosal hypertrophy. Occasionally, when such bony partitions are a cause of localized persistent disease and are inaccessible from the intranasal route, a limited sublabial approach may be indicated for exposure and removal. Clinically and based on research [4], it seems that residual osteitic bony partitions, such as a partially retained infraorbital ethmoid cell, can be a focus for residual inflammation, if not totally resected.

Careful examination of the sinus floor for retained foreign bodies, such as inspissated concretions, dental filling material, or bone chips, should be performed. Instances when this disease is inaccessible through a wide middle meatal antrostomy may require a limited Caldwell-Luc approach or a sublabial maxillary sinus endoscopy. Using the latter, one can inspect and débride the entirety of the sinus cavity. If inspissated material, such as a fungal ball, is evident on the floor of the sinus, the offending material can be removed by lifting it up using the tip of the trocar as a spoon to where it can be accessed by a curved suction through the middle meatal antrostomy.

Failure of mucociliary transport often results from systemic disease, such as cystic fibrosis or Kartagener's syndrome, and is identified by history, laboratory studies, and microscopy. In these situations, deviation from the concept of "FESS" and acceptance of gravity drainage must be practiced. A "megaostium" (ie, one that encompasses most of the medial wall of the maxillary sinus) should be created to allow for copious nasal irrigation with concomitant appropriate head positioning to allow for gravity drainage.

In general, revision maxillary sinus surgery revolves around the principle of opening the flow of secretions by improvement of any factors that play a role in stasis of secretions. The maxillary sinus mucosa is particularly sensitive to the effects of airflow, which can produce significant mucociliary stasis through desiccation. When the maxillary sinus extends significantly medially into the nose, a prior antrostomy has the potential to direct airflow into the maxillary sinus if the residual posterior maxillary sinus wall has not been removed. In this situation, the medially protruding posterior-medial wall should be removed flush with the pterygoid plate, even if an adequate antrostomy already is present. When undertaking primary surgery in a patient with environmental allergies in which the maxillary sinus protrudes medially into the nasal cavity, maintaining a small ostium that protects the posterior maxillary sinus wall from inhaled allergens is preferred. Finally, infected secretions from the frontal or anterior ethmoid sinuses can drain into a maxillary sinus. Treatment in this situation is focused on addressing the frontal/ethmoid disease.

Ethmoid sinus

The ethmoid sinus is central to the other three paranasal sinuses, and most revision sinus surgery includes a total ethmoidectomy to allow complete access to each diseased sinus. In primary chronic rhinosinusitis, surgery is focused toward areas of disease. Although this focus is still the intention of revision surgery, often the entire ethmoid cavity is involved in the disease process with underlying osteitic bone. In such circumstances, the goal of revision surgery is to create a marsupialized cavity, lined by healthy, intact mucosa.

To optimize mucosal healing, resection of as much osteitic bone as is reasonable is necessary. As in primary sinus surgery, the authors advocate dissection low in an anterior-to-posterior direction, across the basal lamella to the sphenoid face, with identification of the skull base in the sphenoid sinus followed by completing the dissection from posterior to anterior. In revision surgery, the skull base provides the second critical landmark after identification of the medial orbital wall and must be identified carefully. This identification is achieved more easily and more safely in the posterior ethmoid or sphenoid sinus. As mentioned earlier, more common findings within the ethmoid cavity during revision surgery are a lateralized middle turbinate, retained uncinate process, failure to remove the uncinate superiorly (persistent recessus terminalis), and residual agger nasi cells. Careful attention to bony lamellar remnants, the use of through cut forceps, and judicious use of the microdébrider help achieve resection of disease, while leaving a mucosal-lined cavity. Sometimes thickened bony lamellae are fractured with a Blakesley forceps, but they usually are not removed with this instrument, so as to minimize the risk of mucosal stripping. Typically, they are teased out, and the mucosal edges are trimmed with the microdébrider. Occasionally, when the bone has become markedly thickened from osteitis, part or much of the revision ethmoidectomy has to be performed with a suction-irrigation drill. Iatrogenic disease also may include a meningocele or encephalocele. In a case in which a skull base dehiscence is identified and a meningocele is suspected, intrathecal injection of fluorescein (0.1 mL of 10% fluorescein mixed with 10 mL of the patient's own CSF) may be considered [20]. The management of skull base defects and CSF leaks is discussed in substantial detail by Bolger and Schlosser elsewhere in this issue.

Sphenoid sinus

Persistent sphenoid sinus disease often is encountered as a result of one of three possibilities: (1) failure to enter the sphenoid at the original surgery, (2) stenosis from inadequate postoperative débridement, or (3) scarring of the

superior turbinate to the face of the sphenoid. Before entering or reentering
the sphenoid sinus, as stated previously, it is advisable to review the radiographic anatomy multiple times in the coronal and axial planes. In addition,
the surgeon should review the course of the optic nerve and carotid artery,
especially if a sphenoethmoid (Onodi) cell is present. The carotid artery is
"clinically dehiscent" in 23% of sphenoid sinuses, and the potential for serious complications in this region is significant (Fig. 7) [21]. When the sphenoid intersinus septum deviates from the midline, it often inserts adjacent to
the carotid artery on the side of deviation. Preoperative diagnosis through
radiologic studies is paramount. When the diagnosis is more firmly established, and risk to surrounding structures is evaluated, multiple approaches
to the sphenoid have been described. Determination of extent of disease and
remaining anatomic landmarks dictates the necessary approach.

The most frequently used approach to the sphenoid sinus for management of sphenoid sinusitis in the setting of chronic rhinosinusitis is transethmoidal. A sphenoidotomy is combined with an ethmoidectomy. Use of
a 0° endoscope is preferred over the 30° endoscope for approaching the
sphenoid because it helps prevent inadvertent superior migration of the
dissection. After complete ethmoidectomy, the sphenoid face, skull base,
and superior turbinate are identified [18,22]. In the presence of severe disease, the last-mentioned landmark may be difficult to identify medially
within the cavity. In some settings, it may be helpful to resect the infe-
rior-posterior portion of the middle turbinate with a backbiter just as
the ground lamella transitions from the horizontal plane to vertical, to expose further the superior meatus and the superior turbinate. Image guidance may be used for confirmation of these landmarks with the
knowledge that accuracy tends to be reduced posteriorly. When the appropriate structures are identified, the inferior one third of the superior turbinate is resected, and the natural ostium of the sinus is identified medially.
The ostium is widened with a j curet, mushroom punch, and rotating Ha-
jek punch. Occasionally, in revision cases, the bone is so thickened that
a diamond burr and suction irrigation drill may be required. In the presence of significant osteitic bone, it is important to create a wide opening,
which extends to the skull base and medial orbital wall. It is important
to remember when entering the sphenoid to stay medial and inferior.
When open, the extent of superior and lateral extension can be appreciated, and the ostium can be enlarged, always feeling behind the bone before resection. In general, at least at a revision procedure, the anterior
face should be taken down to where it is almost flush with the medial orbital wall and the skull base.

The posterior septal branch of the sphenopalatine artery courses along
the inferior face of the sphenoid, approximately 1 to 1.5 cm below the sphenoid ostium. Suction cautery may be required to control bleeding if this
vessel is violated. Postoperatively, resection of scar tissue is important during follow-up examinations to avoid stenosis or restenosis.

The endoscopic transnasal approach may be used in isolated sphenoid disease. This approach is quick and avoids disruption of the anatomy within the ethmoid sinuses. It offers the least total exposure to the sinus of all the approaches, however. The natural ostium of the sphenoid sinus is identified transnasally, medial to the middle and superior turbinates. For this approach, a 0° or 30° endoscope may be used. The natural ostium of the sphenoid sinus is in the sphenoethmoidal recess, at the junction of the superior two thirds and the inferior one third of the superior turbinate. The natural ostia usually can be cannulated in cases of mild disease, and the mushroom punch can be used to widen the ostium. A portion of the superior turbinate should be removed to extend the antrostomy well laterally.

Before the endoscopic era, a transseptal approach was employed most often. It continues to provide the advantage of keeping the surgeon in the midline of the nasal cavity. With the exception of skull base surgery, however, the transseptal approach is rarely used today. Before the endoscopic era, it usually was performed by intraseptal dissection initiated through a hemitransfixion incision. When performed endoscopically, the posterior septum usually is resected transnasally, providing exposure to both sphenoid sinuses.

In the transseptal approach, the midline prominence of the sphenoid sinus appears as the prow of a ship and is removed with chisels and Kerrison rongeurs to enter the sinus itself. Key technical points in using this approach include the need for excellent injections to decrease bleeding in the septal flaps, careful attention to the flaps to prevent tearing, and identification of the sphenoid ostia before entering the sinus. This approach gives extreme wide exposure and still finds favor with surgeons who prefer an operating microscope to an endoscope for work in the sphenoid sinus or behind the sinus for tumor. Additionally, this approach can be used for three-handed and possibly four-handed endoscopic resections.

Frontal sinus

Revision endoscopic frontal sinus surgery requires substantial experience in endoscopic techniques. Adequate visualization of the region requires 45° and sometimes 70° angled endoscopes. In addition to the appropriate angled endoscopes, it is important that the surgeon have available and be familiar with a broad range of angulated through-cut punches and curets, which are necessary to address disease in such a tight anatomic region. Numerous air cells may constitute the frontal recess, including the agger nasi cell, the supraorbital ethmoid cell, frontal sinus cells, interfrontal sinus septal cell, suprabullar cell, frontal bullar cell, and recessus terminalis, complicating the anatomy of the region.

The initial step in frontal recess dissection is identification of the appropriate boundaries and the drainage pathway of the frontal recess. Axial CT scans or scrolling through the image-guided surgery system often helps to determine anterior/posterior and medial/lateral location of the outflow path. Endoscopically, the inferior boundaries of the recess need to be identified. These are laterally the lamina papyracea, medially the insertion of the middle turbinate, anteriorly the nasofrontal beak, and posteriorly the superior extent of the ethmoid bulla. A fine malleable probe can be helpful in palpating the multiple paths under direct visualization for locating the true access to the frontal sinus. The primary approach to the frontal sinus, including the intricate anatomy of the frontal recess, is discussed by Kuhn in substantial detail elsewhere in this issue. Particular attention must be given to understanding and conceptualizing the three-dimensional anatomy of this region from multiplanar CT scans in advance of the surgical procedures and, where possible, identification of the drainage pattern by scrolling through images on a surgical navigation device before the procedure is helpful. In any case, it is important to assess the degree of neo-osteogenesis preoperatively. Marked neo-osteogenesis may make it preferable to avoid the area and the possibility for further regional scarring or may necessitate the use of a 70° angled diamond burr.

A frontal sinus rescue is an extension of the standard endoscopic frontal sinusotomy [23]. In situations in which the middle turbinate has been partially amputated with subsequent scarring to the lateral nasal wall, exposed and osteitic bone often is encountered on the lateral surface of the remnant of middle turbinate when the frontal recess is dissected. In these situations, it is preferable to remove the remainder of the middle turbinate to the skull base carefully, preserving, where possible, the remaining mucosa on the lateral surface. The preserved mucoperiosteal flap can be rotated medially and laid superiorly against the skull base.

Occasionally, a frontal sinus trephine is helpful as an adjunct procedure to view lateral frontal sinus lesions and the frontal recess from above through an endoscopic approach. After creating a trephine, a 2.7-mm or 4-mm endoscope is introduced, allowing an "above and below" approach to frontal sinus lesions. This additional view can aid in clearing the frontal recess of disease. In this situation, a trephine in the anterior wall of the sinus is more useful than a trephine in the floor of the frontal sinus. Other authors have described irrigation through the frontal sinus trephine with colored fluid to help identify the location of the frontal sinus opening when viewed from below endoscopically.

The endoscopic transseptal sinusotomy, sometimes referred to as a Draf III procedure or modified endoscopic Lothrop, creates a large common drainage pathway for the frontal sinuses by removing the superior anterior nasal septum in conjunction with bilateral frontal recess dissection (from orbit to orbit) and removal of the frontal sinus floor bilaterally. The procedure has been described in multiple ways [24–26] and is recommended as a final endoscopic approach before committing the patient to an obliterative procedure [27]. In many cases, unless there is significant pneumatization of the frontal sinus above the nasal septum, a high-speed drill is required, resulting in significant mucosal loss and the probability of postoperative scarring. In evaluating patients for the potential applicability of this approach, it is important to review the anterior-posterior dimensions of the frontal recess and to evaluate the amount of bone that would need to be removed to create a satisfactory opening. Experience dictates that a minimum of 5 mm exists in the anterior/posterior dimension for this approach to be successful. The ability to reduce intranasal and mucosal trauma from the drill has been enhanced by the introduction of 70° suction irrigation drills and by the use of interactive imaging [28]. Even in skilled hands, this operation still carries a risk of CSF leak, however. The surgery can be performed starting medially, through the nasal septum at a point anterior to the anterior attachment of the middle turbinate, or laterally from an open frontal recess. The endoscopic findings are correlated with preoperative CT scans and image guidance. Because of the mucociliary clearance pattern of the frontal sinus, it is imperative to preserve the mucosa of the lateral inferior sinus and recess, as this is the site for physiologic drainage of the sinus. In the midline, working transseptally, the floor of the frontal sinus appears as the prow of a ship, and the frontal sinus is entered from below using a combination of an angled curet and angled drills. During a transseptal frontal sinusotomy, the most anterior portion of the skull base is in the midline, creating a midline ridge that follows the curve of the skull base as it transitions from horizontal to vertical.

When a transseptal frontal sinusotomy is to be performed, it is crucial to discuss with the patient and subsequently perform extensive and meticulous postoperative débridement to keep the newly created common frontal sinus ostium open and ensure mucosolization of the exposed bone.

Postoperative care

Revision surgical patients may require endoscopic follow-up for years if the subsequent chances of recurrence are to be minimized, with careful reevaluation of the medical therapy, based on the endoscopic appearance of the cavity. Additional CT studies also may be required if the original symptoms persist or new symptoms occur, and the cause is not evident on endoscopy. It is easier and more effective to intervene earlier in the disease process with débridement, steroids, and antibiotics than to allow the process to proceed to the point that the patient requires additional revision surgery for removal of hyperplastic or polypoid disease. In the setting of a well-executed surgery and recurrent symptoms, especially loss of olfaction or nasal congestion, anti-inflammatory treatments are often successful. In all situations of medical management, the goal is to minimize oral steroid use and transition to a combination of topical and mechanical treatments as soon as possible. If this transition is done prematurely, however, excessive inflammation is likely to return, and the transition should be based on the endoscopic appearance of the cavity. The authors use a burst and prolonged taper of oral steroids leading to every-other-day dosing before the burst is discontinued. Repeat imaging with CT typically is not required, assuming that a patent cavity was achieved at surgery. A repeat CT scan is warranted, however, for persistent symptoms that cannot be explained by endoscopy and may show undissected cells.

Summary

Patients with recurrent chronic sinusitis after prior surgical intervention pose a particular challenge to the otorhinolaryngologist. Establishing a correct diagnosis is the first step and requires review of the original presurgical symptoms and imaging; review of the more recent symptoms and images; and reevaluation of environmental, general, and local host factors that may contribute to persistent disease. Although primary chronic rhinosinusitis is typically a medical disease, postsurgical persistent disease may result directly from iatrogenic causes, requiring early surgical revision. Even in this setting, however, proper preoperative medical therapy is essential.

Diagnostic evaluation should include meticulous endoscopic evaluation and appropriate radiologic studies. CT typically is required in the coronal and axial planes and ideally is performed using a computer-assisted surgical navigation protocol and with reconstructions in the sagittal plane, allowing for "scrolling" through the altered anatomy and conceptualizing the surgical issues at hand.

When the decision to undergo revision surgery is made, the patient and the physician need to comprehend the rigorous and prolonged schedule of postoperative care and débridements that may be required for long-term success. Appropriate surgical technique emphasizing mucosal preservation and complete dissection must be adhered to. The surgeon must be aware that bony thickening is likely to be present and to make the dissection significantly more difficult than in the primary case. Medical management and endoscopic surveillance postoperatively is continued until a stable cavity is achieved.

References

[1] Senior BA, Kennedy DW, Tanabodee J, et al. Long-term results of functional endoscopic sinus surgery. Laryngoscope 1998;108:151.

[2] Kennedy DW, Senior BA, Gannon FH, et al. Histology and histomorphometry of ethmoid bone in chronic rhinosinusitis. Laryngoscope 1998;108:502.

[3] Moriyama H, Yanagi K, Ohtori N, et al. Healing process of sinus mucosa after endoscopic sinus surgery. Am J Rhinol 1996;10:61.

[4] Perloff JR, Gannon FH, Bolger WE, et al. Bone involvement in sinusitis: an apparent pathway for the spread of disease. Laryngoscope 2000;110:2095.

[5] Parsons DS, Stivers FE, Talbot AR. The missed ostium sequence and the surgical approach to revision functional endoscopic sinus surgery. Otolaryngol Clin North Am 1996;29:169.

[6] Bhattacharyya N. Computed tomographic staging and the fate of the dependent sinuses in revision endoscopic sinus surgery. Arch Otolaryngol Head Neck Surg 1999;125:994.

[7] Zeifer B. Sinusitis: postoperative changes and surgical complications. Semin Ultrasound CT MR 2002;23:475.

[8] Brown CL, Graham SM. Nasal irrigations: good or bad? Curr Opin Otolaryngol Head Neck Surg 2004;12:9.

[9] Faden H, Britt M, Epstein B. Sinus contamination with *Pseudomonas paucimobilis*: a pseudoepidemic due to contaminated irrigation fluid. Infect Control 1981;2:233.

[10] Bolger WE, Kuhn FA, Kennedy DW. Middle turbinate stabilization after functional endoscopic sinus surgery: the controlled synechiae technique. Laryngoscope 1999;109:1852.

[11] Chiu AG, Vaughan WC. Revision endoscopic frontal sinus surgery with surgical navigation. Otolaryngol Head Neck Surg 2004;130:312.

[12] Fried MP, Moharir VM, Shin J, et al. Comparison of endoscopic sinus surgery with and without image guidance. Am J Rhinol 2002;16:193.

[13] Koele W, Stammberger H, Lackner A, et al. Image guided surgery of paranasal sinuses and anterior skull base—five years experience with the InstaTrak-System. Rhinology 2002;40:1.

[14] Hurst RW, Judkins A, Bolger W, et al. Mycotic aneurysm and cerebral infarction resulting from fungal sinusitis: imaging and pathologic correlation. AJNR Am J Neuroradiol 2001;22:858.

[15] Chu CT, Lebowitz RA, Jacobs JB. An analysis of sites of disease in revision endoscopic sinus surgery. Am J Rhinol 1997;11:287.

[16] Ramadan HH. Surgical causes of failure in endoscopic sinus surgery. Laryngoscope 1999;109:27.

[17] Musy PY, Kountakis SE. Anatomic findings in patients undergoing revision endoscopic sinus surgery. Am J Otolaryngol 2004;25:418.

[18] Orlandi RR, Lanza DC, Bolger WE, et al. The forgotten turbinate: the role of the superior turbinate in endoscopic sinus surgery. Am J Rhinol 1999;13:251.

[19] Richtsmeier WJ. Top 10 reasons for endoscopic maxillary sinus surgery failure. Laryngoscope 2001;111:1952.

[20] Lanza DC, O'Brien DA, Kennedy DW. Endoscopic repair of cerebrospinal fluid fistulae and encephaloceles. Laryngoscope 1996;106:1119.

[21] Kennedy DW, Zinreich SJ, Hassab MJ. The internal carotid artery as it relates to endonasal sphenoethmoidectomy. Am J Rhinol 1990;4:7.

[22] Bolger WE, Keyes AS, Lanza DC. Use of the superior meatus and superior turbinate in the endoscopic approach to the sphenoid sinus. Otolaryngol Head Neck Surg 1999;120:308.

[23] Citardi MJ, Javer AR, Kuhn FA. Revision endoscopic frontal sinusotomy with mucoperiosteal flap advancement: the frontal sinus rescue procedure. Otolaryngol Clin North Am 2001;34:123.

[24] Draf W. Endonasal micro-endoscopic frontal sinus surgery: the Fulda concept. Oper Tech Otolaryngol Head Neck Surg 1991;2:234.

[25] Gross WE, Gross CW, Becker D, et al. Modified transnasal endoscopic Lothrop procedure as an alternative to frontal sinus obliteration. Otolaryngol Head Neck Surg 1995;113:427.

[26] McLaughlin RB, Hwang PH, Lanza DC. Endoscopic trans-septal frontal sinusotomy: the rationale and results of an alternative technique. Am J Rhinol 1999;13:279.

[27] Weber R, Draf W, Kratzsch B, et al. Modern concepts of frontal sinus surgery. Laryngoscope 2001;111:137.

[28] Chandra RK, Schlosser R, Kennedy DW. Use of the 70-degree diamond burr in the management of complicated frontal sinus disease. Laryngoscope 2004;114:188.

ELSEVIER
SAUNDERS

Otolaryngol Clin N Am
39 (2006) 437–461

OTOLARYNGOLOGIC
CLINICS
OF NORTH AMERICA

An Integrated Approach to Frontal Sinus Surgery

Frederick A. Kuhn, MD[a,b]

[a]Georgia Nasal & Sinus Institute, 4750 Waters Avenue, Suite 112, Savannah, GA 31404, USA
[b]Department of Otolaryngology, University of North Carolina, Chapel Hill, NC, USA

The frontal sinus has been recognized as a problem since Ambrose Pare first described a white sticky substance oozing from it during skull trephination in 1564 [1]. Although Lettre originally described frontal sinus trephine in 1704 [1], Ogston reported the first external surgical procedure on the frontal sinus in 1884 [1]. Since then, there have been a myriad of frontal sinus procedures developed to deal with chronic frontal sinusitis. These procedures range from the destructive Riedel procedure, in which the anterior frontal sinus table is removed, to the Sewell-Boyden and McNaught procedure, which reconstructs the frontal sinus drainage pathway by rotating a nasal mucosal flap into an enlarged frontal ostium [2–4]. Others include:

- The Lynch procedure [5], which requires an external incision and removes the lateral frontal recess wall;
- The Lynch procedure as modified by Neel, McDonald and Facer [6], which removes less of the lateral frontal recess wall, but also requires an external incision
- The Lothrop procedure [7,8], which requires an external incision and removes interfrontal sinus septum, frontal sinus floor, and upper nasal septum
- The intranasal approaches as championed by Van Alyea and others in the early 1900s
- The Draf drill-out procedures [9] and the endoscopic modified Lothrop procedure described by May [10] and Gross [11]
- Frontal sinus obliteration, which became the standard in the last half of the 20th century [12]

Most, if not all of these procedures, had and still may have their place. The array of available operations, however, varies from the sublime to the deforming. To say the least, the list is confusing as to which procedure is the best. Some of the procedures are of historical interest only, while others still have utility in the correct situation. It became apparent that a logical system of organization needed to be brought to this problem. To that end, the most useful procedures were organized into a comprehensive integrated approach to frontal sinus surgery. It begins with the least invasive and progresses to the most invasive procedure in a step-by-step fashion, which can be applied as needed. The selection of procedure is governed by the patient's disease, anatomy, and the surgeon's skill. The least invasive procedure that can be used should be attempted first, and then, if more is needed, other procedures can be added, either at the same sitting or in subsequent revisions.

The overriding principle is to restore frontal sinus physiologic function and to preserve all normal structures, particularly the middle turbinate, which provides the medial frontal recess support. This may require only a procedure as simple as relieving anterior ethmoid disease or one as complex as reconstructing and repneumatizing an obliterated frontal sinus. The surgeon's inability to perform a less invasive, more physiologic procedure is not a reason to perform a greater, more invasive or destructive procedure.

Frontal sinus anatomy and physiology

The most important concepts to master in understanding the frontal sinus are:

1. Contrary to long-held popular concepts, the drainage pathway, not the frontal sinus, is the primary cause of chronic frontal sinusitis.
2. The frontal recess, an inverted funnel shaped space, not a tubular shaped duct, connects the sinus to the anterior ethmoid region and is the controlling area in frontal sinus drainage.
3. Frontal recess obstruction is the primary cause of chronic frontal sinusitis, not the sinus.
4. Frontal sinus ciliary beat pattern and therefore mucus flow is up the interfrontal sinus septum, lateral across the frontal sinus roof, and then medial over the frontal sinus floor to the ostium (Fig. 1).

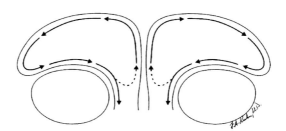

Fig. 1. Frontal sinus mucociliary flow and clearance pattern.

5. Mucus clearance out of the sinus is active by ciliary action down the lateral aspect of the frontal recess, whether it is directly down the medial orbital wall, or over the medial aspect of a frontal recess cell, such as an agger nasi cell.

6. During frontal recess dissection, if these cell walls are removed up to their attachment at the medial orbital wall, and the frontal recess and medial orbital wall mucosa is preserved intact, ciliary mucus clearance will continue uninterrupted.

7. If this mucus membrane is damaged or removed, the sinus may not function properly after healing. As Moriyama demonstrated in 1996, pseudostratified, ciliated columnar epithelium does not regenerate well after being stripped off of bone [13].

8. Only 40% to 60% of the frontal sinus mucus is swept out of the frontal sinus on any given circuit of the mucus around the interior of the frontal sinus. The other 60% to 40% recirculates around the sinus [14]. Messerklinger also demonstrated that the mucus may sweep down into the frontal recess and then back up into the frontal sinus, potentially taking bacteria, fungus, or debris with it into the sinus.

9. The funnel-shaped frontal sinus connection to the anterior ethmoid sinus, is a potential space, not an open funnel or a tubular-shaped duct as taught in the 19th and 20th centuries [15]. The three-dimensional frontal recess first was described by Killian in 1896 [16] and later extensively discussed by Schaeffer [17], Kaspar [18], and Van Alyea [19]. Van Alyea gave an extensive description of the cells pneumatizing and potentially obstructing this space, the frontal sinus drainage pathway [20,21].

10. One must master frontal recess anatomy to safely adopt the endoscopic frontal recess approach [22,23] and the other frontal sinus procedures developed from it. Building on Van Alyea's work, a series of articles has described each of the frontal recess cells anatomically and radiographically and their potential contribution to frontal sinus obstruction [24–28].

11. The surgeon is ready to become trained in the specialized techniques of frontal sinus surgery, only after understanding this anatomy and how external ethmoidectomy, drilling in the frontal recess, and middle turbinate collapse or resection, may alter or compromise frontal sinus drainage.

The integrated frontal sinus surgery approach

Box 1 lists the most useful procedures arranged in order from least to most invasive. The question remains as to which is the right surgical procedure for a particular patient. The general rule is to choose the least invasive procedure with which the surgeon is comfortable and which will accomplish the task. Additional procedures then may be employed as the situation

---

Box 1. The integrated approach to frontal sinus surgery

Endoscopic frontal sinuplasty
Endoscopic frontal sinusotomy [22,23]
Frontal sinus rescue procedure [29,30]
Above and below approach (trephine and endoscopic) [31]
Modified intranasal endoscopic Lothrop (without drill)
Modified intranasal endoscopic Lothrop (with drill) [9–11]
Above and below approach (osteoplastic flap and endoscopic)
    [31]
Osteoplastic flap with frontal sinus obliteration [12]
Frontal sinus unobliteration [32]
Frontal sinus cranialization

---

dictates. More specifically, most cases can be managed endoscopically (Box 2). If the case is started endoscopically and the disease cannot be reached or the anatomical problem solved, however, additional more aggressive procedures can be added in a stepwise fashion. As an example, a trephine could be added to the endoscopic approach, the procedure converted to an extended frontal sinus rescue (FSR) or to a modified Lothrop, or the case rescheduled for an open procedure. Each of the integrated approach techniques will be discussed.

Box 2. Frequency of procedures in the integrated approach for frontal sinus surgery

Endoscopic frontal sinuplasty
Endoscopic frontal sinusotomy—90% of cases
Frontal sinus rescue procedure—80 procedures in 9 years
Above and below approach (trephine and endoscopic)—less than
    1/year
Modified intranasal endoscopic Lothrop (without drill)—three in
    3 years
Modified intranasal endoscopic Lothrop (with drill)—four in
    14 years
Above and below approach (osteoplastic flap and endoscopic)
Osteoplastic flap with frontal sinus obliteration—five in 10 years
Frontal sinus unobliteration—40 in 15 years
Frontal sinus cranialization—0%

Endoscopic frontal sinusotomy

Endoscopic frontal sinusotomy [22,23] is the natural extension of the intranasal headlight techniques advocated a century ago, but with the addition of far better imaging and visualization. It has stood the test of time, as compared with its ancestral procedure, because there is long-term follow-up to demonstrate its longevity. The CT scan, extremely clear optics, and high-resolution video cameras provide the diagnostic tools and the visibility to perform these delicate intranasal procedures. In addition, there is proof that thin axial sinus CT sections, even with a single-slice scanner, will not expose the patient to added cataract risk [33]. Siller's study provided surgeons with the ability to obtain sagittal sinus CT reconstructions and thin axial sections for diagnosis and use with image-guided surgery computers, before helical scanners were available and at a time when neuroradiologists were reluctant to do thin axial sections for fear of producing cataracts.

Clear, highly detailed sagittal reconstructions from thin axial CT sections have improved dramatically the surgeon's ability to understand the patient's frontal recess anatomy by looking at it laterally. Therefore, the surgeon is able to ascertain the anatomical reason for frontal recess/frontal sinus obstruction and determine the best surgical approach to the problem. This is demonstrated by Fig. 2, the coronal views of an opaque frontal recess without an obvious cause. The sagittal reconstruction in Fig. 2, however, demonstrates the persistent ethmoid bulla lamella just posterior to the opaque frontal recess, which needs to be removed. The endoscopic pictures in Fig. 3 illustrate the clear skull base posterior to the bulla lamella and the polyps filling the frontal sinus drainage pathway anterior to the lamella. The solution to this mechanical problem is the targeted removal of the residual ethmoid bulla lamella.

The combination of delicate endoscopic techniques, new frontal sinus instruments designed to allow the surgeon to work further up in the frontal

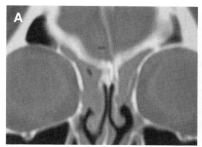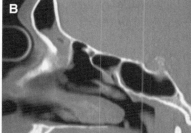

Fig. 2. (A) Coronal CT shows obstructed frontal recess with no obvious etiology. (B) Sagittal CT reconstruction demonstrates residual ethmoid bulla lamella, causing frontal recess obstruction.

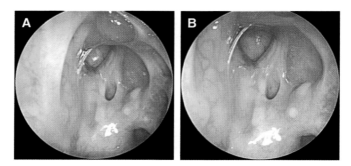

Fig. 3. (*A*) Endoscopic view demonstrates polyps anterior to bulla lamella. (*B*) Endoscopic view demonstrates normal skull base posterior to bulla lamella.

sinus, and image-guided surgery, has extended the surgeon's ability and reduced the need to use some of the other techniques. Many patients who might have required the combined above and below (endoscopic and trephine) approach 10 years ago now can be managed endoscopically. The patient in Fig. 4 presented with chronic frontal sinusitis and pain following sinus surgery several years before. He had a large residual Type III frontal cell obstructing the right frontal sinus (see Fig. 4). Although the middle meatus preoperatively appears to be normal with a 0° telescope, the 70° telescope reveals polyps filling the frontal recess (see Fig. 4. This case was managed strictly endoscopically using Kuhn-Bolger (Karl Storz) frontal sinus instruments in 1996. The patient's frontal sinus remains widely patent and functional 9 years after surgery (see Fig. 4).

There are several principles important to frontal recess surgery. Dissection should be performed from posterior to anterior and from medial to lateral to avoid damaging the thinnest areas of bone surrounding the frontal recess. The posterior frontal recess table is commonly very thin and subject to penetration with subsequent cerebrospinal fluid (CSF) leak. The same pertains to the medial posterior frontal recess, bounded by the lateral cribriform plate lamella. The other principle is to preserve all frontal recess mucus membrane, because sinus mucus membrane does not regenerate over bare bone with normal cilia.

The ethmoidectomy should be performed first and the frontal recess approached from posterior along the skull base. As previously noted in discussing the agger nasi cell [13], its two walls that can be removed are the posterior and medial walls. This anatomical relationship extends to the frontal cells also, and in essence means that the frontal sinus not only drains over the medial and posterior walls, but that it can be approached the same way from below (ie, posterior and medial). Consequently, once the ethmoid dissection is complete, the frontal recess cells can be removed with frontal sinus punches (Karl Storz) (Fig. 5) or fractured from posterior to anterior and from medial to lateral with frontal recess curettes (see Fig. 5). The fragments

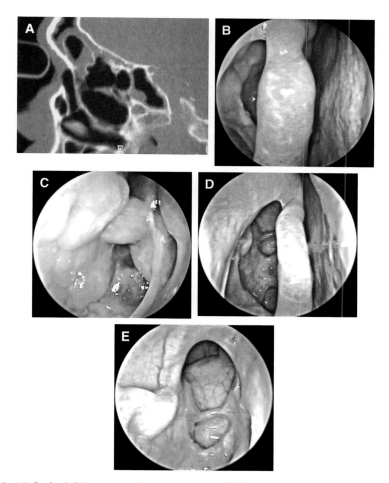

Fig. 4. (*A*) Sagittal CT reconstruction shows a type III frontal cell remaining after previous sinus surgery. (*B*) Endoscopic view of the right middle meatus with a 0° telescope (*C*) Endoscopic view of the right meddle meatus with a 70° telescope. (*D*) Postoperative endoscopic view of the right middle meatus with a 0° telescope. (*E*) Postoperative endoscopic view of the right middle meatus with a 70° telescope.

then are removed gently with giraffe forceps (see Fig. 5) or by using short bursts of a joint shaver/tissue debrider. The process is repeated as needed until the frontal ostium is clear. Frontal ostium seekers (see Fig. 5) are used to retrieve small pieces of bone, which may remain in the frontal sinus or recess.

The frontal ostium can be stented or left alone depending on how widely open it is and how well the mucosa drapes over the edge of the frontal ostium. Soft flexible silastic stents rather than semirigid stents should be used as reported by Neel and Lake in their research on frontal sinus stents in dogs

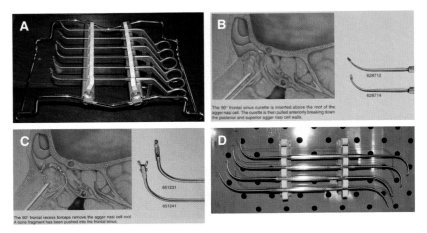

Fig. 5. (*A*) Frontal sinus punches. (*B*) Frontal ostium curettes. (*C*) Frontal sinus 90° giraffe. (*D*) Frontal sinus seekers (Courtesy of Karl Storz, Culver City, California.)

[34]. They demonstrated that semirigid stents induced circumferential scaring and osteoneogenesis at the frontal ostium in their dog frontal sinus experiments. Soft 0.01 inch thick silastic sheeting cut and rolled into a T shape makes an excellent frontal sinus stent (Fig. 6).

Endoscopic frontal sinuplasty

The rightful place of sinuplasty is first as the least invasive of all procedures listed. This procedure, however, just introduced at the American Academy of Otolaryngology meeting in September 2005, needs to be discussed after endoscopic frontal sinusotomy, because it requires the same

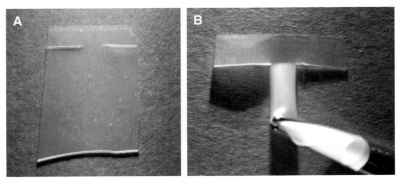

Fig. 6. (*A*) Cut silastic sheeting for frontal sinus stent. (*B*) Silastic sheeting rolled into configuration for a frontal sinus stent.

anatomical understanding, as does standard endoscopic frontal sinusotomy. Frontal sinuplasty may find its place as a stand-alone procedure besides being used in conjunction with endoscopic frontal sinusotomy. The author is in the early stages of its use and has found it to be, at the very least, a surprisingly simple and straight-forward method of identifying the frontal sinus drainage pathway and identifying the air cell walls compromising it, which need to be removed.

When used as a stand-alone procedure, it provides a straight-forward means of cannulating the frontal sinus (Fig. 7) and dilating the drainage pathway (see Fig. 7) without damaging the mucociliary clearance mechanism. It accomplishes this by pushing the medial agger nasi cell wall laterally and the ethmoid bulla lamella posteriorly (see Fig. 7). The balloon does this without crushing the agger nasi cell completely and obstructing its drainage pathway. When performed with endoscopic ethmoidectomy, it is counterintuitive to leave any cell walls around the frontal ostium. Upon realizing that the natural ciliary clearance mechanism has not been disturbed, however, it makes more sense. When viewed endoscopically several months postoperatively, even though the remaining cell walls around the frontal ostium still seem as though they should have been removed. The frontal ostium looks healthy and is functional (Fig. 8).

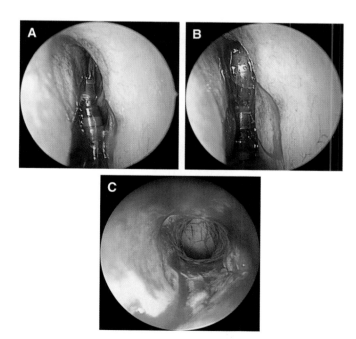

Fig. 7. (*A*) Uninflated sinuplasty balloon in the left frontal recess. (*B*) Inflated sinuplasty balloon in the left frontal recess. (*C*) Dilated frontal sinus drainage pathway immediately after balloon sinuplasty. (Courtesy of Acclarent, Menlo Park, California; with permission.).

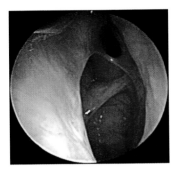

Fig. 8. Healed right frontal recess 10 weeks after balloon sinuplasty. The bony posterior wall of the ostium is the remaining bulla lamella. The preserved uncinate process is anterior and inferior to the ostium.

The procedure is performed with a series of instruments under fluoroscopic control by endoscopically placing a 70° or 90° guiding cannula (Fig. 9) into the upper middle meatus and passing the guide wire through it up into the frontal sinus. The placement of the guiding cannula is improved by using image guidance to identify the entrance to the frontal recess, which is usually medial against the middle turbinate and further posterior than expected. If the guide wire meets resistance, its position is checked easily with fluoroscopic snapshots, rather than use continuous fluoroscopy, and the guiding cannula is repositioned. This saves radiation exposure. Once the wire is in the sinus (Fig. 10), a balloon catheter is passed over it into the frontal sinus, its position checked fluoroscopically, and the balloon is inflated to dilate it fully. The balloon can be observed dilating the ostium fluoroscopically as seen in see Fig. 10. As the balloon is inflated, the ends fill first, because the ostium creates a pinch effect in the middle. As bone is fractured around the ostium, the balloon fills completely (see Fig. 10). This may take as little as four to six atmospheres of pressure. One observation is that greater pressure may create more and longer-lasting

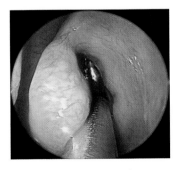

Fig. 9. Guiding cannula in the upper middle meatus at the entrance to the frontal recess (Courtesy of Acclarent, Menlo Park, California, with permission.).

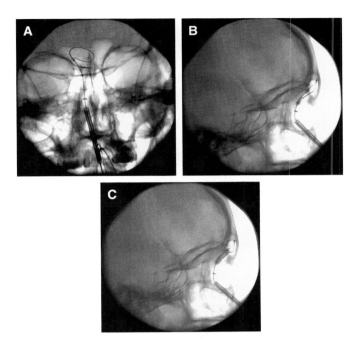

Fig. 10. (*A*) This fluoroscopic image demonstrates the guide wire in right frontal sinus. The guiding cannula can be seen at lower part of image with the marker at its tip and guide wire protruding from it. The two black dots on the guide wire mark the ends of the uninflated balloon in place over the guide wire. (*B*) Fluoroscopic image of partially inflated balloon over guide wire in frontal sinus. (*C*) Fluoroscopic image of fully inflated balloon in frontal sinus drainage pathway.

mucosal edema. The balloon may be repositioned one or more times over the length of the drainage pathway as needed.

Fig. 7 shows the left frontal sinus roof seen through the left frontal ostium immediately after dilation with a 7 mm balloon. The agger nasi cell wall was pushed laterally without compromising its lumen.

Fig. 8 is a right frontal sinus opening 10 weeks after sinuplasty with a 5 mm balloon. It is patent and has an estimated diameter of 3 mm. Several cell wall remnants may be seen below the opening, which were not removed after the standard endoscopic ethmoidectomy was performed. Anterior is the uncinate process and posterior is the ethmoid bulla lamella. The frontal sinus drainage pathway is functional and open.

This procedure may be used alone for isolated frontal sinus disease or in conjunction with sinuplasty of the maxillary and sphenoid sinuses. It also may be used in combination with endoscopic ethmoidectomy in a hybrid procedure, because sinuplasty is not adapted to ethmoid surgery. Its benefit is to identify and treat the frontal sinus more quickly and accurately with less risk of mucus membrane damage.

Frontal sinus rescue procedure

FSR [29,30] was designed for those patients whose middle turbinate had been amputated previously and whose middle turbinate remnant had lateralized. Many of these patients might otherwise have been obliterated or subjected to a drill-out procedure. The concept of the frontal sinus rescue is to reopen the frontal recess and devise a way to keep the frontal ostium open. The procedure involves identifying the frontal recess, opening it, and then resecting the nasal mucosa overlying the superior middle turbinate remnant. Next, the frontal recess mucosa is dissected off of the turbinate remnant carefully, and the residual middle turbinate bone is resected to the skull base. The last step is to create a flap from the preserved medial frontal recess mucosa and turn it up onto the roof of the nasal vault. This creates a circular frontal sinus ostium continuous with the medial orbital wall mucosa, but with a rectangular flap breaking up the circumference of the circle, superiorly (Fig. 11).

The patient in Fig. 12 is a 37-year-old man who had four endoscopic sinus surgeries in 10 years and then four semirigid stent placements over the previous year. He presented with the stents in place and with continuing staphylococcal infections. As can be seen in Fig. 12, both middle turbinates had been amputated, and tubular silastic stents, the same size as the frontal openings are in place. Fig. 12 also shows the sagittal reconstruction, demonstrating a horizontal plate of bone posterior to the stent and a loculated area above it. The stent was removed, as seen in Fig. 12, revealing an opening the size of the stent into the infected frontal sinus. The posterior

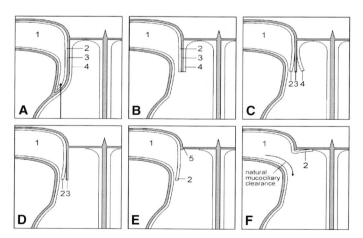

Fig. 11. The steps in the frontal sinus rescue procedure. The frontal recess is identified and penetrated; then the nasal mucosa and frontal recess mucosa are dissected free of the bony middle turbinate remnant. This bone and the nasal mucosa (from the medial surface of the middle turbinate) are resected at the skull base, and the frontal recess mucosal flap is rotated up onto the nasal vault roof, where it stays by capillary action. The new frontal ostium may be stented depending on the surgeon's assessment (*1*, frontal sinus; *2*, mucoperiosteal flap; *3*, bony stub of middle turbinate; *4*, mucosa on medial surface middle turbinate).

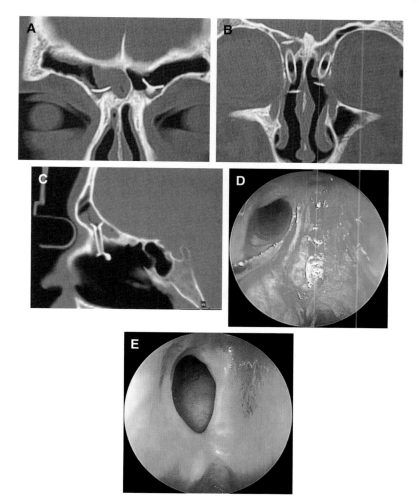

Fig. 12. (*A*) Coronal sinus CT shows semirigid stents in infected frontal sinuses. The stents are the same size as the ostium. (*B*) Coronal sinus CT demonstrates that the middle turbinates have been resected. (*C*) This sagittal CT view demonstrates a bony plate behind right stent. (*D*) Endoscopic view of the right frontal ostium immediately after stent removal. (*E*) Endoscopic view of the right frontal ostium, 3 years after FSR.

plate of bone was removed, and a medial flap was constructed and turned up onto the nasal vault roof. Fig. 12 also demonstrates the new frontal sinus opening 3 years after surgery.

Extended frontal sinus rescue

The ExFSR was developed for patients with an intact middle turbinate, but with a collapsed frontal recess, which is so narrow that it will not respond to the standard endoscopic technique. The procedure involves cutting a narrow channel up the middle turbinate to its superior attachment at the skull base (Fig. 13). Once this is accomplished, one proceeds as with the FSR. The remaining middle turbinate commonly attaches itself to the lateral nasal wall below the new frontal ostium, so that the frontal sinus drains directly into the nose above the middle turbinate and the reformed middle meatus.

The patient in Fig. 14 had a collapsed frontal recess and underwent a left extended frontal sinus rescue procedure. He returned for right frontal sinus surgery, and because the left frontal ostium was small, it was revised at the same sitting. Fig. 14 also demonstrates the new ostium above the reattached middle turbinate. Additionally, Fig. 14C shows the nasal mucosa dissected off of the frontal recess mucosa and the frontal recess mucus membrane flap cut and turned over onto the nasal roof.

Above and below technique (frontal sinus trephine & endoscopic) [31]

This technique is used for frontal sinus lesions or cells that cannot be reached from below, but can benefit from a bimanual approach somewhat short of an osteoplastic flap. This may be used for small frontal sinus osteomas, CSF leaks, or large frontal cells beyond the reach of the frontal ostium. The endoscopic procedure is performed as described, and an eyebrow incision is made. The incision is moved up the forehead and medially over the frontal sinus. The periosteum is incised, and a 4 mm cutting burr is used to make an anterior table trephine. It is important to make the trephine through the

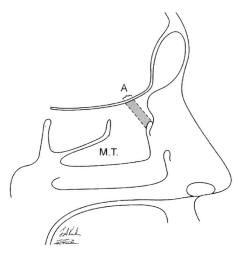

Fig. 13. This diagram shows the extended frontal sinus rescue procedure, which includes a channel cut into middle turbinate up to the skull base.

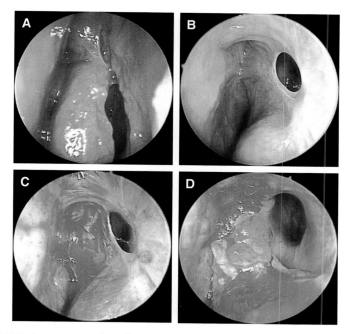

Fig. 14. (*A*) Endoscopic view of a collapsed left frontal recess that did not respond satisfactorily to the standard endoscopic approach. (*B*) Endoscopic view of the left middle turbinate reattached to lateral nasal wall below new frontal ostium. (*C*) Endoscopic view of revision sinus rescue demonstrates nasal mucosa separated and removed from frontal recess mucosa in preparation for flap creation. (*D*) Endoscopic view of frontal sinus rescue shows the frontal recess mucosal flap turned onto the nasal roof.

anterior table, rather than through the floor because of the angle required to see down into the frontal recess. When operating, the 30° telescope is positioned or rested on the edge of the trephine, so that the view is down into the frontal sinus. The instruments are passed into the sinus through the trephine below the telescope (Fig. 15). The telescope may be passed into the sinus if necessary to inspect something inside the sinus, but it is not practical to have telescope and instruments in the sinus at the same time. At the conclusion of the procedure, the wound is sutured with a 3-0 absorbable suture, and adhesive strips are applied to the skin.

Two patients are demonstrated here, the first with a frontal recess osteoma, which was fractured off of its attachment, but was too large to extract through the frontal ostium (Fig. 16). An anterior frontal sinus table trephine measuring 5 × 10 mm was created, so the osteoma could be pushed up into the frontal sinus and drilled in half. It then was dropped down through the frontal ostium and removed. The eyebrow healed with no scar, and no evidence of bony forehead defect was noted. The frontal recess was healed, and there was no recurrence on CT when last seen, 7 years after surgery (see Fig. 16).

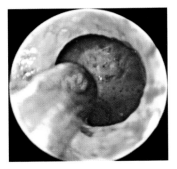

Fig. 15. Endoscopic view of an instrument passed through the trephine (through a 30° telescope positioned on bony rim of trephine).

The second patient had a previous osteoplastic frontal sinus procedure without obliteration by means of a coronal incision, but the lateral frontal sinus cell was missed, because it was peripheral to the bone flap cut. The cell was accessed through an eyebrow incision and a 4.5 mm anterior table trephine (Fig. 17). The intervening cell wall was removed through the trephine (see Fig. 17), and the cell is connected widely to the right frontal sinus as seen on the endoscopic photograph (see Fig. 17). Seven years postoperatively, there has been no recurrence of the partition separating the lateral cell from the frontal sinus.

Endoscopic modified Lothrop (Draf III)

The original external Lothrop described in 1914 [7,8] was an interesting operation that did not achieve lasting popularity. Lothrop's concept was to create a large common frontal sinus opening into the nose. He approached the frontal sinus externally from one side, removing the interfrontal sinus septum, the medial frontal sinus floor, and the upper nasal septum.

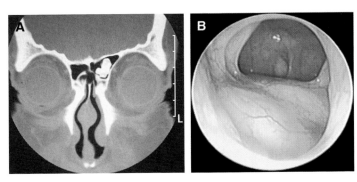

Fig. 16. (A) Coronal sinus CT of a left frontal recess osteoma. (B) Endoscopic view of the left frontal ostium, 7 years after endoscopic removal of osteoma.

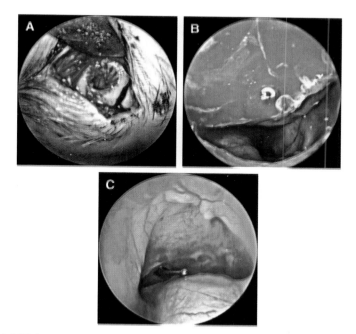

Fig. 17. (*A*) Right eye brow incision with frontal sinus trephine partially completed, and a bone cut medial to trephine from previous osteoplastic frontal sinus procedure. (*B*) Endoscopic view through the trephine down to frontal recess, demonstrating that the crescent-shaped partition separating the lateral cell from the frontal sinus has been removed. (*C*) Endoscopic view of a frontal ostium seeker passed into the frontal sinus through the trephine, as seen looking up through the frontal recess.

He did not remove the mucus membrane of the upper medial orbital walls and therefore did not interfere with frontal sinus drainage.

The shortcoming of the currently used endoscopic modification of this procedure is that to perform it, a drill is employed to remove the agger nasi region up into the frontal sinus and to drill across the midline joining the two sides. The drilling in the agger nasi region usually destroys the lateral frontal recess mucus membrane. This mucus membrane specifically is the mucus transport mechanism out of the frontal sinus. Consequently, this puts the frontal sinus at risk for mucociliary clearance failure and for the opening to stenose.

Lanza [35] described a trans-septal approach to frontal sinusotomy in 2001, which avoids damage to the lateral frontal recess mucosa, an important improvement over the modified intranasal Lothrop procedure.

Just making a large opening is no guarantee that the frontal sinus problem will be solved, as evidenced in Fig. 18. This patient illustrates the need for continued follow-up and clinical thinking about the underlying disease processes. She had a true external Lothrop procedure 10 years earlier, but presented with an infected, painful frontal sinus. Cultures and other laboratory work

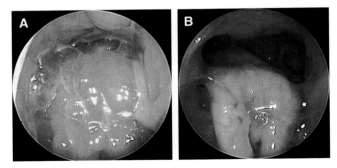

Fig. 18. (*A*) Endoscopic view of infection and polyps in a true external Lothrop sinusotomy, demonstrating that ostium size alone is not enough to guarantee patency. (*B*) Endoscopic view of same patient shows impact of treatment with systemic prednisone. Fungus and eosinophils were found on pathologic smear, and IgE was elevated.

ultimately demonstrated an infection with *Pseudomonas aueriginosa* and allergic fungal sinusitis. She responded to antibiotics and prednisone (see Fig. 18), and when her allergic fungal sinusitis is under control, the frontal sinus functions well, because the lateral frontal recess mucus membrane remains intact.

Modified Lothrop without drill [36]

In some patients, the bone of the medial frontal sinus floor and the interfrontal sinus septum can be removed with frontal sinus punches without using a drill, thereby preserving the maximum frontal recess mucus membrane and normal frontal sinus mucus clearance. The patient illustrated here presented with the middle and superior turbinates and the upper nasal septum removed from her nose, yet she remained chronically infected. Fig. 18 demonstrates her sinuses at their worst and best. After trying to control her disease for 10 years, it was discovered while revising her ethmoid roof that the medial frontal sinus floor and interfrontal sinus septum could be removed with frontal sinus punches, while preserving her lateral frontal ostium mucus membrane. Consequently, a modified intranasal Lothrop was performed, and the frontal sinus mucociliary clearance mechanism was preserved (Fig. 19). The area in the right frontal sinus, which continually sequestered bacteria, was in a very narrow cleft behind the right orbit, which could not be accessed or obliterated. This area is now more open and accessible to office treatment, and the ciliary pathway out of the sinus is preserved. As a consequence, her infections have decreased dramatically. This technique offers a possible means of improving the outcomes of the intranasal modified Lothrop procedure.

Above and below (osteoplastic and endoscopic) [31]

This procedure provides unparalleled access to the frontal recess. It is the procedure of choice for frontal sinus tumors, such as inverting papilloma,

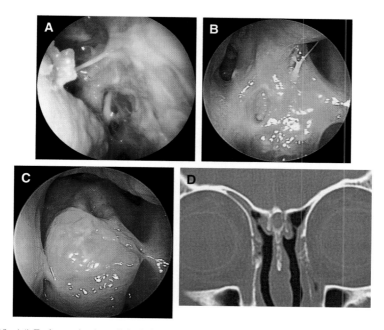

Fig. 19. (*A*) Endoscopic view of the left nasal roof demonstrates frontal ostia covered with pus. (*B*) Endoscopic view shows the right and left frontal ostia before revision modified endoscopic Lothrop procedure with punches. (*C*) Endoscopic view of the same area after modified endoscopic Lothrop with punches.

so that the sinus may be imaged postoperatively. It is also the procedure of choice for unobliteration, because it gives the best opportunity to completely remove whatever material was used to obliterate the sinus originally and to open the frontal recess. It also provides access to the farthest extent of the sinus to reconnect distant isolated pockets of mucus membrane to the frontal recess by custom fitting thin-sheet silastic stents to the pattern of the frontal sinus. These stents have a frontal recess extension that can be rolled and passed down through the frontal recess into the ethmoid sinus for later removal of the entire stent. When the frontal sinus work is finished, the stents are positioned in the sinus and the flap replaced. Frontal sinus stents in this case commonly are left in place for 6 to 12 months. If the sinus becomes chronically infected, the stent likely will develop a biofilm that will keep the sinus infected. If this happens, the stent eventually will need to be removed to allow the infection to resolve.

Frontal sinus obliteration [12]

There are practical contraindications to frontal sinus obliteration. The author has demonstrated in unpublished data that frontal sinus obliteration may fail, because the mucus membrane was not all removed despite careful drilling of the bone. The author has revised five frontal sinus obliteration patients whose bony frontal sinus walls had been drilled and their frontal sinus obliterated with fat. Four patients presented 2 to 15 years after obliteration with acute frontal sinusitis. The first was an 18-year-old patient who developed a draining fistula from the frontal sinus to the left upper eyelid within 2 years of obliteration and eventually underwent five corneal transplants before the sinus was controlled. The fifth presented with chronic sinusitis, frontal pain, and decreased vision in his left eye. A massive mucocele involving the frontal sinus and the left supraorbital ethmoid cell was found, which had eroded the entire left orbital roof, depressed the globe, and compromised vision (Fig. 20). All five patients' frontal sinuses were found to be entirely relined with mucus membrane and filled with mucopus. Other patients in the series had mucus membrane pockets around the periphery of the obliterated sinus under the anterior frontal sinus table, peripheral to the bone flap. Others failed because of missed supraorbital ethmoid cells. Still others recurred at the frontal recess, where mucosal disease was trapped between the obliterated frontal sinus above and an unoperated frontal recess below. The contraindications are related to the inability to know whether all mucus membrane has been removed from the bony frontal sinus walls. These contraindications are: missing posterior frontal sinus table bone, missing orbital roof bone, extensive supraorbital ethmoid cell pneumatization, frontal sinus tumor, and allergic fungal sinus.

The reasoning behind these contraindications is that one cannot be certain the mucus membrane is removed completely while preparing the frontal sinus for obliteration, even by drilling the bone. Consequently, one definitely cannot be certain of removing the mucus membrane from the dura or the periorbita, which cannot be drilled, in the event that the posterior table or orbital roof is eroded. In each case, frontal sinus mucosa is adherent to soft tissue, either to the dura or to the periorbita.

In the case of extensive supraorbital ethmoid pneumatization, the illustrations almost speak for themselves. The spaces at the farthest extent of the cells are either inaccessible or too narrow to get a drill into. It makes much more sense to remove the frontal recess obstruction and repneumatize the cells (Fig. 21).

When dealing with fungus or tumor, such as inverting papilloma, one also can never be certain of complete removal. Therefore, it is far better postoperatively to be able to image an air-containing frontal sinus and detect recurrence than to deal with the vagaries of imaging an obliterated sinus.

From 1950 until the 1990s, the standard operation taught for treating chronic frontal sinusitis was either osteoplastic frontal sinus obliteration or the Lynch external fronto–ethmoidectomy. In many places, the focus was on the frontal sinus. The frontal recess and the ethmoid sinuses often were overlooked, as demonstrated by patients who still have complete ethmoid opacification after frontal sinus obliteration. This may have been

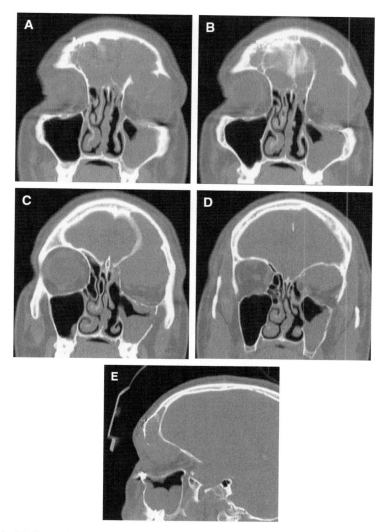

Fig. 20. (*A*) Coronal sinus CT image of an obliterated frontal sinus with a mucocele eroding left orbital roof. (*B*) Coronal sinus CT shows a large left supraorbital ethmoid cell lateral to frontal sinus with orbital roof erosion and globe displacement caused by mucocele expansion into the orbit. (*C*) More posterior coronal sinus CT image demonstrates the full extent of mucocele. (*D*) Coronal sinus CT shows mucocele expansion into posterior orbit with displacement of the globe, and stretching of the optic nerve. (*E*) Sagittal CT reconstruction demonstrates that the entire orbital roof has been eroded. Note the degree of mucocele protrusion into orbit.

because of a lack of adequate radiologic imaging, because the sinus CT scan only came into use in the mid 1980s. Now that sinus imaging and anatomical understanding have improved, osteoplastic frontal sinus obliteration is no longer the standard of care and has assumed a much lesser role. It is not an operation that should be performed with any frequency, because it is

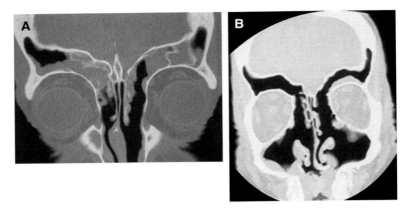

Fig. 21. (A) Coronal sinus CT of an obstructed supraorbital ethmoid cell. (B) Coronal sinus CT (obtained after revision endoscopic frontal sinusotomy shows that the supraorbital ethmoid cell is now clear.

destructive and may lead to long-term complications. It now is relegated to last-resort status. As a rule, if there is any question about whether all of the frontal sinus mucus membrane can be removed, obliteration should not be performed. Again, the surgeon's lack of ability to perform a lesser procedure is not a reason or an indication to obliterate the frontal sinus. For instance, obliteration is not the first choice of operation in the instance of amputated or lateralized middle turbinate with frontal recess and frontal sinus obstruction. There are certain instances in which this is the only alternative, such as when there is no possibility of re-establishing a connection between the sinus and the anterior ethmoid sinus. There are definitely instances in which it should not be obliterated.

Frontal sinus unobliteration [32]

When frontal sinus obliteration has failed, the sinus must be re-explored, either endoscopically to open the frontal recess/ostium, or through an osteoplastic flap or by a combined approach. If the osteoplastic flap is performed, the opportunity presents itself to reverse the obliteration or unobliterate the sinus. The primary symptom of frontal obliteration failure is persistent, unremitting hard frontal pain. Not every patient with chronic frontal pain has a frontal sinus mucocele, and not every patient with a frontal sinus mucocele has pain; however, a significant percentage of patients do. When all conservative methods have failed to account for or to control the pain, it is often necessary to re-explore the sinus. This generally is done through a coronal incision for cosmetic purposes, which also preserves sensory innervation to the forehead.

Failure falls into several categories:

- Frontal sinuses that are relined completely with mucus membrane, filled with mucus or pus and with no evidence of fat

- Mucus or pus-filled mucus membrane pockets around the periphery of the sinus far removed from the frontal recess
- Frontal recess mucoceles trapped between intrinsic obstruction below and the obliterated sinus above
- Mucopyoceles in obstructed unrecognized supraorbital ethmoid cells

As noted previously, it is notoriously difficult to predict whether all mucus membrane has been removed, even when the anterior and posterior tables have been drilled. One does not need to revise many frontal sinus obliteration patients to begin suspecting the wisdom of ever performing this procedure. After revising over 40 of these patients, the author has come to the conclusion that it is not a good operation. In the best of hands, the results are problematic, and in the worst of cases, the operation may not even have been indicated in the first place.

When unobliterating a frontal sinus, the primary task is to reconnect the peripheral mucosalized areas to a functional frontal ostium. This involves ensuring that there is no persistent obstruction to these pockets of mucosa around the sinus (usually beyond the bone cut and under the anterior frontal sinus table) and then laying a 0.01 inch-thick silastic template onto the posterior sinus table, which extends out into these pockets. A large flap on the inferior aspect of the template is rolled and passed down through the frontal ostium to act as a stent, so that every part of the sinus and outflow tract is covered and protected from synechiae formation. This stent/template is left in place for 1 year or longer, as long as it does not become infected. If it becomes infected, it eventually needs to be removed to clear up the infection; however, if removed too early, the sinus may fill with scar tissue and wall off areas of mucosa again.

One might ask then, why not just reobliterate the sinus instead of going to this much trouble? The response is, for the same reason that it did not work the first time. How can anyone be certain of removing all of the mucus membrane the second time? One of the problems with this issue is that rarely does one see his or her own failures. One may see other's failures, but no one otorhinolaryngologist does enough obliterations or practices long enough to see all of his or her own failures. Consequently, otorhinolaryngologists simply assume everything is just fine.

The second major task is recreating a functional connection to the nose or anterior ethmoid sinus. There are clearly instances in which the Lothrop procedure, which is very straightforward when the frontal sinus is open, is the best solution to ensuring a patent ostium. In other instances, the endoscopic frontal sinusotomy is best.

Frontal sinus cranialization

This procedure is mentioned only to condemn it. It is performed commonly by neurosurgeons or plastic surgeons who have little understanding of the ramifications associated with leaving sinus mucus membrane in a closed space. Its primary utility is in frontal sinus or skull fractures or after tumor resections. The problem is the possibility of intracranial regeneration of mucus membrane producing an intracranial mucocele, which would be even more difficult to remove. The risk is increased by the methods used to remove all of the mucus membrane. One technique commonly used is to cauterize away all of the mucus membrane. If there truly is no possible way to salvage the posterior frontal sinus table, an otorhinolaryngologist should be involved in drilling away the last vestiges of the mucus membrane if there is no other choice than to cranialize the sinus. If possible, the dura should be repaired, the frontal sinus salvaged, and the frontal recess opened widely to provide clear, permanent frontal sinus drainage. For those concerned about the safety of these alternatives, cranializing the frontal sinus does not make it safe, and obliterating it does not make it safe; therefore, using safety as an argument is fallacious.

Summary

In conclusion, although many procedures devised for the frontal sinus are useful, most chronic frontal sinus cases can be successfully treated endoscopically. A scheme of organization has been applied to most of the useful procedures, so that they are arranged in order of increasing complexity and invasiveness. They thus are integrated into a whole concept, which then can be applied progressively to any patient's situation in a logical order as required by the anatomy, the disease process, and the surgeon's skill. The reader is reminded that lack of ability to perform less invasive procedures is not justification for performing greatly more invasive ones. The day of major invasive frontal sinus surgery as the standard of care for chronic frontal sinus disease is long past.

References

[1] Anderson CM. External operation on the frontal sinus: causes of failure. Arch Otolaryngol 1932;15:739–45.
[2] Sewall EC. The operative treatment of nasal sinus disease. Ann Otol Rhinol Laryngol 1935; 44:307.
[3] McNaught RC. A refinement of the frontoethmosphenoid operation: a new nasofrontal pedicle flap. Arch Otolaryngol 1936;23:544.
[4] Boyden GL. Surgical treatment of chronic frontal sinusitis. Ann Otol Rhinol Laryngol 1952; 61:558.
[5] Lynch RC. The technique of a radical frontal sinus operation which has given me the best results. Laryngoscope 1921;31:1.
[6] Neel HB, McDonald TJ, Facer GW. Modified lynch procedure for chronic frontal sinus disease: rationale, technique, and long term results. Laryngoscope 1987;97:1274.
[7] Lothrop HA. Frontal sinus suppuration. Ann Surg 1914;49:937–57.
[8] Lothrop HA. Frontal sinus suppuration with results of new operative procedure. JAMA 1915;65:153–60.
[9] Draf W. Endonasal microendoscopic frontal sinus surgery: the Fulda concept. Operative Techniques in Otolaryngology/Head and Neck Surgery 1991;2:234–40.

[10] May M. Frontal sinus surgery: endonasal endoscopic osteoplasty rather than external osteoplasty. Operative Techniques in Otolaryngology/Head and Neck Surgery 1991;2:226–31.
[11] Gross CW, Zachmann GC, Becjer DG, et al. Follow-up University of Virginia experience with the modified Lothrop procedure. Am J Rhinol 1997;11:49–54.
[12] Goodale RI, Montgomery WW. Technical advances in osteoplastic frontal sinusectomy. Arch Otolaryngol 1964;79:522–9.
[13] Moriyama H, Yanagi K, Ohtori N, et al. Healing process of sinus mucosa after endoscopic sinus surgery. Am J Rhinol 1996;10:61–6.
[14] Messerklinger W. On the drainage of the normal frontal sinus of man. Acta Otolaryngol 1967;63:176–81.
[15] Mosher HP. Transactions American Laryngological Association 1912;34:25–39.
[16] Killian G. Zur anatomie der Nase menschlicher Embryonen. Arch Laryngol Rhinol 1896;4:1–45.
[17] Schaeffer JP. The genesis, development and adult anatomy of the nasofrontal region in man. Am J Anat 1916;20:125–45.
[18] Kasper KA. Nasofrontal connections: a study based on one hundred consecutive dissections. Arch Otolaryngol 1936;23:322–43.
[19] Van Alyea OE. Ethmoid labrynth: anatomic study with consideration of the clinical significance of its structural characteristics. Arch Otolaryngol 1939;29:881–901.
[20] Van Alyea OE. Frontal cells. Arch Otolaryngol 1941;34:11–23.
[21] Van Alyea OE. Frontal sinus drainage. Ann Otol Rhinol Laryngol 1946;55:267–78.
[22] Kuhn FA. Operative techniques in chronic frontal sinusitis: the endoscopic frontal recess approach. Operative Techniques in Otolaryngology/Head and Neck Surgery 1996;7:222–9.
[23] Kuhn FA, Javer AR. Primary endoscopic management of the frontal sinus. Otolaryngol Clin North Am 2001;34:59–75.
[24] Kuhn FA, Bolger WE, Tisdal RG. The agger nasi cell in frontal recess obstruction: an anatomic, radiologic and clinical correlation. Operative Techniques in Otolaryngology/Head and Neck Surgery 1991;2:226–31.
[25] Bent JP, Cuilty-Siller C, Kuhn FA. The frontal cell in frontal sinus obstruction. Am J Rhinol 1994;8:185–91.
[26] Owen RG, Kuhn FA. The supraorbital ethmoid cell. Otolaryngology Head and Neck Surgery 1997;116:254–61.
[27] Merritt R, Bent JP, Kuhn FA. The intersinus septal cell. Am J Rhinol 1996;10:299–302.
[28] Kuhn FA. Surgery of the frontal recess. In: Kennedy DW, Bolger WE, Zinreich J, editors. Diseases of the sinuses: diagnosis and management. Hamilton (Ontario, Canada): B.C. Decker; 2001. p. 281–301.
[29] Citardi MJ, Javer AR, Kuhn FA. Frontal sinus rescue procedure. Otolaryngol Clin North Am 2001;34:123–32.
[30] Kuhn FA, Javer AR. Frontal sinus rescue (FSR) procedure: early experience and follow-up. Am J Rhinol 2000;14:211–6.
[31] Bent JP, Spears RA, Kuhn FA, et al. Combined endoscopic intranasal and external frontal sinusotomy (the above and below approach to frontal sinusotomy: alternatives to obliteration). Am J Rhinol 1997;11:349–54.
[32] Javer AR, Sillers MS, Kuhn FA. Unobliteration of the frontal sinus. Otolaryngol Clin North Am 2001;34:193–210.
[33] Sillers MJ, Kuhn FA, Vickery CL. Radiation exposure in paranasal sinus imaging. Otolaryngology Head and Neck Surgery 1995;112:248–51.
[34] Neel HB, Whicker JH, Lake CF. Thin rubber sheeting in frontal sinus surgery: animal and clinical studies. Laryngoscope 1976;86:524–36.
[35] Lanza DC, McLaughlin RB, Hwang PH. The five-year experience with endoscopic transseptal frontal sinusotomy. Otolaryngol Clin North Am 2001;34:139–52.
[36] Dubin MG, Kuhn FA. Endoscopic modified Lothrop (Draf III) with frontal sinus punches. Laryngoscope 2005;115:1702–3.

ELSEVIER
SAUNDERS

Otolaryngol Clin N Am
39 (2006) 463–473

OTOLARYNGOLOGIC
CLINICS
OF NORTH AMERICA

Perioperative Care for Advanced Rhinology Procedures

Richard R. Orlandi, MD[a],*, Peter H. Hwang, MD[b]

[a]Division of Otolaryngology–Head and Neck Surgery, Center for Therapeutic Biomaterials,
The University of Utah, 50 North Medical Drive, 3C120, Salt Lake City, UT 84132, USA
[b]Department of Otolaryngology–Head and Neck Surgery, Stanford University,
801 Welch Road, Palo Alto, CA 94305-5739, USA

Successful outcomes in rhinologic surgery require careful endoscopic interventions, not only in the operating room, but also in the perioperative setting. In particular, meticulous postoperative care is essential to successful outcomes. Nasal endoscopy during the postoperative period affords the surgeon the opportunity to debride the cavity and prevent scarring, maintain patent ostia, and tailor medical therapy. Although superior intraoperative technique does not obviate the need for attentive postoperative care, many aspects of preoperative and intraoperative care can influence a patient's postoperative care and ultimate clinical outcome. This article reviews aspects of wound healing and perioperative care that can optimize surgical patency and clinical outcome.

Sinus wound healing

To achieve success in endoscopic sinus surgery, a familiarity with concepts of wound healing is essential. Wound healing is a complex and orderly sequence of events that involves various cell types and subcellular signals. Despite the fact that sinus surgery is performed so widely, little is known about wound healing in the paranasal sinuses, and most current information on epithelial wound healing comes from epidermal studies [1]. Although

Dr. Orlandi is a consultant for and has a significant financial interest in Carbylan BioSurgery, Incorporated.
* Corresponding author.
E-mail address: richard.orlandi@hsc.utah.edu (R.R. Orlandi).

general principles are likely similar, findings in epidermis should be applied to sinus mucosal wound healing with caution.

Inflammation is the first of the three phases of wound healing, followed by proliferation and remodeling [2]. The inflammatory phase involves the influx of macrophages and other cells from the circulation and the subsequent release of cytokines and mediators [3–5]. Oxygen-free radicals are generated as a part of the inflammatory reaction, particularly by neutrophils that are present in the early phases of inflammation. These radicals can cause further tissue damage. Following the inflammatory phase, proliferation of new tissue takes place. Within 4 days of the injury, a loose connective tissue matrix containing hyaluronan, fibronectin, and collagen is present. Inflammatory cells continue to provide signals that regulate the healing processes at this stage, such as angiogenesis, fibroplasia, and re-epithelialization. Unlike epidermal injuries, where hair follicles, glands, and other skin appendages provide the primary source for new epithelial cells after wounding, respiratory epithelium appears to regenerate mostly from undifferentiated basal cells from adjacent noninjured areas [6]. As inflammation and proliferation subside, remodeling of the wound takes place. The extracellular matrix changes, with hyaluronan and other glycosaminoglycans diminishing, while elastin and proteoglycan deposition increases. These remodeling changes evolve over months, pointing out the need for prolonged postoperative endoscopic evaluation.

Although healed sinus mucosa may appear identical to nontraumatized mucosa grossly, important differences are seen at a microscopic level, including marked fibrosis and decreased glands. Cilial abnormalities also are seen, including complex and edematous cilia and fewer than normal cilia per unit area [7,8]. Ciliary function also is impaired following mucosal regeneration, with slowed and disorganized mucus transport [9]. These facts underscore the importance of minimizing mucosal injury during surgery. Common sense dictates that the minimal amount of mucosal wounding results in the minimal risk of scarring and mucosal dysfunction.

Preoperative considerations

Proper preoperative medical therapy must be put in place to reduce inflammation and resulting vasodilation that can hamper visualization during surgery [10]. For example, careful preoperative endoscopy is necessary to make an accurate diagnosis and to guide preoperative anti-inflammatory and antimicrobial medical therapy. Antibiotics, preferably culture-directed, may be effective when infection is present. Topical corticosteroids may help reduce inflammation also. In cases of significant preoperative inflammation, such as nasal polyposis, systemic corticosteroids may be indicated. Nonsteroidal anti-inflammatory medication and herbal supplements that may impair coagulation should be stopped before surgery to minimize bleeding that may impair visualization.

Intraoperative considerations

Meticulous technique in the operating room often can minimize and simplify the postoperative care needs of the patient. Intraoperatively, attention to mucosal preservation enables quicker and more complete return of normal mucociliary clearance. In surgery for chronic rhinosinusitis, these goals are accomplished best with meticulous surgical technique directed toward restoring the patency of the natural sinus ostia while minimizing tissue trauma. Even during ablative procedures such as endoscopic neoplasm resection, preservation of healthy mucosa is desirable to maintain as much residual sinonasal function as possible.

At the time of surgery, vasoconstriction with topical and injected medications is essential to preserve visualization, allowing for more meticulous and thorough dissection. The authors prefer oxymetazoline spray just before surgery, followed by injections of lidocaine with epinephrine intraoperatively. Topical vasoconstriction is applied repeatedly throughout the surgery as needed, using neurosurgical cottonoids soaked in oxymetazoline or 1:1000 epinephrine. The use of topical concentrated epinephrine is avoided in pediatric and geriatric populations, or in those with poorly controlled hypertension [11]. During surgery, mucosal removal must be minimized. Cutting instruments should be employed whenever possible to avoid leaving bare areas of bone. Demucosalized areas have been theorized to result in osteoneogenesis and perpetuation of inflammation [12]. In addition, large areas of missing mucosa tend to heal without organized ciliary movement, hampering the return of normal sinus function [7,9].

Mucosal disruption where two surfaces are in contact often will lead to annealing of the surfaces during wound healing, even if the degree of disruption is minimal. This phenomenon is most common between the lateral surface of the middle turbinate and the lateral nasal/ethmoid wall. The significance of a synechia in this region depends on its extent. At best, it may be filmy and may only span the middle meatus without narrowing it. Although nonobstructive, this type of scar band still can have a negative impact by preventing placement of an endoscope farther posteriorly, thus compromising the ability to evaluate the rest of the sinuses. More serious sequelae may develop if the scar band contracts during the healing process, lateralizing the middle turbinate. Scar contracture in this critical anatomic zone may lead to maxillary and frontal ostial obstruction and mucosal apposition within the ethmoid cavity. Even in the absence of frank adhesions, the apposition of two mucosal surfaces can lead to perpetuation of inflammation through impaired mucus clearance [13].

Preventing middle turbinate synechiae starts with atraumatic endoscopic technique. In general, all scopes and instruments should be passed carefully through the middle meatus without abrading or contusing the surrounding mucosa (Fig. 1). Collateral injury to adjacent mucosa not only causes unnecessary bleeding that may compromise visualization, but also may create raw surfaces for synechia formation. When approaching the narrow middle meatus or ethmoid cavity, consideration should be given to performing a septoplasty to gain wider access [14].

Another important technical consideration is complete removal of the uncinate process during maxillary antrostomy and anterior ethmoidectomy. This maneuver limits the tissue that can bridge medially from the lateral nasal wall.

Leaving bone and mucosal fragments within the sinuses also can compromise postoperative results and increase the need for postoperative care. Devitalized bone elements can perpetuate inflammation after surgery, and trapped mucosal fragments can lead to mucocele formation. This is especially important in the narrow and relatively unforgiving confines of the frontal recess. Even if the frontal sinus is not explored, stray fragments of bone or mucosa from an anterior ethmoidectomy can block the frontal sinus outflow and lead to iatrogenic frontal sinusitis [15].

The most extensive skull base tumor resection and the most limited anterior ethmoidectomy should conclude with a thorough endoscopic evaluation of the dissection margins to make sure that scar-promoting elements are removed or minimized. At the conclusion of the endoscopic procedure, careful suctioning, and, if necessary, irrigation of the sinuses should be employed to ensure removal of all fragments. The position of the middle turbinate also should be assessed for its propensity to lateralize. If the stability of the middle turbinate is in question, numerous methods to keep the middle turbinate

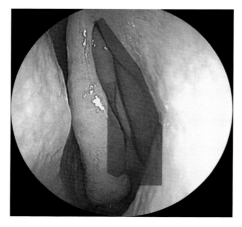

Fig. 1. Left middle meatus. Shaded areas of mucosa are at risk for abrasion and subsequent synechia formation. Great care should be used in passing instruments past these areas.

medialized may be employed, including packing or stenting and suture medialization [16]. Such meticulous care and foresight in the operating room can reduce the need to address undesirable sequelae during the postoperative period.

Postoperative care goals

The purpose of postoperative care following endoscopic rhinologic procedures is to maintain the anatomic patencies achieved during surgery. Postoperative care rarely can compensate for a poor surgical technique, but it can preserve the results of good surgical technique.

Endoscopic debridement is one of the mainstays of postoperative care. The purpose of this technique is to remove potential scar-forming elements, preserve ostial patency, and remove early scar bands. Aggressive debridement does not necessarily promote mucosal healing and may in fact disrupt it [17]. Nevertheless, gentle debridement may be beneficial secondarily by promoting the delivery of topical medication. Eliminating old blood and mucus removes reservoirs of inflammatory mediators and potential media for bacterial growth. Mechanical disruption of fibrin deposits is also important in preventing scar formation. This is especially important in advanced frontal sinus procedures where drilling of bone leaves substantial demucosalized areas. Crusting in these areas may be significant and can lead to ostial closure if left unattended.

Removal of debris within the sinuses also allows for a thorough endoscopic examination. Surgery is an invasive process that exacerbates rather than relieves sinus inflammation in the first days and weeks postoperatively. The speed and degree to which this inflammation resolves varies from patient to patient. This may reflect the individual's own genetic make-up, environment, or nutritional status, but it also likely reflects the various underlying contributors to sinus inflammation [18]. Because of the variability of sinus inflammation and return to normal function, frequent observations of the surgical cavity are necessary to guide appropriate medical therapy.

Current postoperative care strategies

In reviewing strategies for postoperative care, one must recognize that there is no cookbook approach. Patient care must be individualized to achieve maximum benefit. What follows is a general outline, but departures from it likely will be necessary based on patient needs and physician preferences.

Packing and irrigation

Packing typically is placed to control postoperative hemorrhage. It has the potential advantage of filling the ethmoid cavity and diminishing the amount of debris that can accumulate [19]. In general, it is tolerated poorly by patients, however, and is not necessary to prevent postoperative bleeding complications [11]. Moreover, substantial bleeding can occur at the time of packing removal, and oozing may persist afterwards. The ability of nasal packing to limit crusting in the ethmoid cavity therefore may be limited. Newer forms of dissolvable packing may offer significantly greater comfort for patients. Care must be taken, however, to vigilantly debride any nonresorbed residual material, because retained fragments of packing may be associated with local inflammation [20].

Saline irrigation can be helpful in minimizing crusting in the ethmoid cavity. Whether the saline is isotonic or hypertonic is probably less important in the immediate postoperative period than the mechanical effect of the irrigation. In the authors' experience, pulsatile dental irrigating systems have a propensity for promoting *Pseudomonas* infections of the sinuses, likely because of the difficulty in cleansing the apparatus. A simple irrigation bottle or bulb that is easy to keep clean may be most beneficial in the early postoperative period. Likewise, using bottled saline solutions or making a solution with distilled or boiled water should be encouraged to minimize contamination of the sinuses.

Medical therapy

Medical therapy to limit sinus inflammation and prevent bacterial infection of retained secretions is instituted immediately following surgery. When purulence is present at the time of surgery, antibiotics are given based on the Gram's stain and culture results. Otherwise, antibiotics effective against common sinus pathogens are employed. Some evidence indicates macrolide antibiotics may inhibit inflammation by downregulation of the NFκB pathway, similar to corticosteroids, giving them an additional advantage in the postoperative period [21]. The role for antifungal therapy in the postoperative period remains undefined until evidence for its indication and efficacy can be validated by rigorous clinical trials.

Systemic corticosteroids also may be indicated in the postoperative period, particularly in cases of severe inflammation such as nasal polyposis. These typically are given as a taper regimen, with 30 mg of prednisone per day given in the first few days after surgery, tapering down to 10 mg/d by the first postoperative visit. From that point onward, the taper is modified based on the degree of inflammation seen endoscopically. Topical nasal steroid sprays, which will form the mainstay of prolonged medical therapy, typically are restarted during the first postoperative week.

Endoscopic debridement

As with any intervention, endoscopic debridement begins with counseling the patient about the procedure and his/her expectations. Topical anesthesia and vasoconstriction are delivered initially by spraying. It may be necessary to reapply the spray after obstructive crusts are removed or to topically deliver additional medicine with a cotton applicator. Phenylephrine mixed with tetracaine or lidocaine can be used topically and often obviates the need for topical cocaine and its attendant substance control issues. Local injection of anesthetics is rarely necessary but should be considered when topical application is insufficient.

After achieving sufficient anesthesia, debridement of dried mucus and blood from the ethmoid sinuses is performed. Great care must be taken to avoid stirring up additional bleeding, which will diminish the efficacy of the debridement and may require additional intervention at the next visit. Any scar bands or synechia that are present are divided and resected sharply. Obstructive fibrinous debris or exudate should be cleared to prevent progression to mature cicatrix. Additional material in the frontal, sphenoid, and maxillary sinuses typically can be removed with suction but may require removal with endoscopic forceps. Once the cavity is debrided completely, an assessment of the mucosal inflammation is made to guide medical therapy. Ostial patency also is assessed, particularly in the frontal recess. Frontal sinus stenosis can be addressed by resecting any developing scar contracture or by dilating the ostium [15].

Rarely a patient cannot tolerate debridement under local anesthesia. In these cases where the inability to debride and examine the cavity may negatively impact the success of the surgery, the endoscopic debridement can be done in the operating room under sedation, or, if necessary, general anesthesia.

Instrumentation

Proper instrumentation is essential for adequate postoperative care. Nasal telescopes with the angles used during surgery must be available to visualize the sinuses postoperatively. At a minimum, this typically means 0° and 30° telescopes. When frontal sinus surgery is performed, 45° or 70° nasal telescopes also must be available. An adequate light source is necessary to illuminate the cavity, which often contains old blood that reflects less light than the mucosal surface. A camera and monitor afford the patient and family a before and after view of the sinuses and assist them in understanding the need for the debridement and can be helpful, although not essential.

Suctioning is a mainstay of debridement, and both straight (Frazier) and curved canula are necessary (Fig. 2). Straight and 45° upbiting grasping forceps are the workhorse instruments for crust removal in the ethmoid cavity. Although bayonet-shaped forceps can be used, Blakesley-type forceps are more precise and more easily manipulated alongside a nasal telescope. Similarly shaped through-cutting forceps and a sickle knife are also necessary to sharply cut or resect scar bands (Fig. 3).

Frontal sinus surgery necessitates the presence of curved-necked instruments for debridement postoperatively. A 90° angled curette is useful in

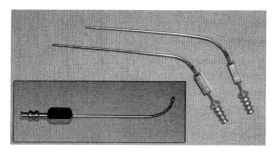

Fig. 2. Straight and curved suction cannulae used in office debridement following endoscopic surgery.

gently freeing crusts within the frontal recess, which then can be removed with grasping forceps, either vertically or horizontally opening. Through-cutting frontal sinus forceps are necessary to deal with scar bands that may form in the frontal recess (Fig. 4).

Postoperative schedule

The timing and frequency of visits are variable, depending on the patient's degree of postoperative inflammation and scarring, their compliance with postoperative medications and instructions, and their response to medical therapy. In the authors' practices, a patient's first postoperative visit generally occurs 1 week following surgery. Following debridement of all operated sinuses and a thorough endoscopic examination, the patient's medical therapy is adjusted as needed. Most patients typically can be seen in another 2 weeks thereafter, although some may need to be seen earlier (especially critical frontal cases), while others can wait longer. Endoscopic debridements and examinations continue every 1 to 3 weeks until the patient is on a stable medical regimen, and the sinus healing and inflammation have stabilized. In the authors' experience, most patients will require about three

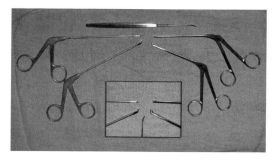

Fig. 3. Both grasping and through cutting Blakesley-type forceps and straight and 45° upturned varieties are useful. A sickle knife is useful for cutting synechia.

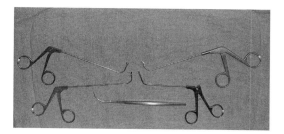

Fig. 4. Curved neck forceps for debriding the frontal recess. Both through cutting and grasping instruments are available that open front to back and side to side. A curved curette is also very useful in the frontal recess.

postoperative visits, although some physicians have reported a routine of up to seven visits postoperatively [22]. It should be stressed that the number of required visits should be based on an individual patient's medical necessity, not on a national average, although such statistics likely will apply to the average physician's practice overall.

After the immediate postoperative period

Postoperative care does not end 2 months after endoscopic sinus surgery. Patients with chronic rhinosinusitis require ongoing monitoring for disease recurrence or worsening. Biochemically and histologically, wound healing following surgical intervention may continue for 6 months to 1 year postoperatively [1]. Chronic mucosal inflammation may abate quite slowly and often incompletely. Patient visits including nasal endoscopy every 3 months are common for the first year postoperatively. In the absence of symptomatic worsening, patients may be seen semiannually or annually thereafter. It should be remembered, however, that inflammatory changes typically can be seen endoscopically before the patient becomes symptomatic [23]. This underscores the need for continual monitoring of this chronic disease. Patients who have undergone endoscopic resection of a skull base neoplasm also require routine endoscopic follow-up to monitor for recurrence.

Future directions

Individual variations in wound healing and inflammation following sinus surgery mandate an individualized approach. At this point, few prognostic factors for favorable wound healing in the sinuses have been identified; thus, it is difficult to predict which patient will have a better surgical outcome. However, as these prognostic indicators become elucidated, physicians may have the opportunity to modulate wound healing to the patient's benefit. One promising lead is the discovery of metalloproteinase-9/gelatinase-B as a marker for wound healing quality [24]. The concentration of this protein, common in the inflammatory and wound healing response, has been found to be highly correlated with the quality of healing during the initial 6 months following surgery. It may be possible to predict, monitor, and influence healing quality following surgery by using MMP-9 and other markers as guides.

Topical delivery of wound-modulating compounds also may play a future role in the postoperative phase of sinus surgery. Retinoic acid has been found to promote epithelial regeneration in an animal model [25]. Mitomycin C has been shown to reduce ostial narrowing in an animal model but has had limited success in human trials, likely because of delivery issues [26–29]. Sustained delivery of these compounds and growth factors may improve their efficacy, and this is possible using therapeutic biomaterials [30,31]. Corticosteroid- and antibiotic-eluting biomaterials also may improve the outcome for patients. Appropriate biomaterials that do not worsen the inflammatory reaction already present may promote epithelialization and speed wound healing and lead to better outcomes following surgical intervention [32,33].

Summary

A superior postoperative outcome begins with meticulous intraoperative technique, leaving sinus cavities with minimal mucosal trauma and no bone and mucosal fragments. The goal of postoperative care is to preserve the surgical patency achieved at the conclusion of surgery. Normal wound healing processes can compromise this through scarring and inflammation. Attentive, thorough, and individualized postoperative care maximizes the patient's chance of a successful outcome. As understanding of sinus wound healing increases, and improved delivery devices and biomaterials are developed, the potential to further improve future outcomes will increase.

References

[1] Watelet JB, Bachert C, Gavaert P, et al. Wound healing of the nasal and paranasal mucosa: a review. Am J Rhinol 2002;16(2):77–84.
[2] Kirsner RS, Eaglestein WH. The wound healing process. Dermatol Clin 1993;11:629–40.
[3] Branski RC, Verdonlini K, Rosen CA, et al. Markers of wound healing in vocal fold secretions from patients with laryngeal pathology. Ann Otol Rhinol Laryngol 2004;113:23–9.
[4] Savla U, Appel HJ, Sporn PH, et al. Prostaglandin E2 regulates wound closure in airway epithelium. Am J Physiol Lung Cell Mol Physiol 2001;280:L421–31.
[5] Kenyon NJ, Ward RW, McGrew G, et al. TGF-beta1 causes airway fibrosis and increased collagen I and III mRNA in mice. Thorax 2003;58:772–7.
[6] Inayama Y, Hook GE, Brody AR, et al. The differentiation potential of tracheal basal cells. Lab Invest 1998;58(6):706–71.
[7] Benninger MS, Schmidt JL, Crissman JD, et al. Mucociliary function following sinus mucosal regeneration. Otolaryngol Head Neck Surg 1991;105(5):641–8.
[8] Toskala E, Rautiainen M. Electron microscopy assessment of the recovery of sinus mucosa after sinus surgery. Acta Otolaryngol 2003;123(8):954–9.

[9] Min YG, Kim IT, Park SH. Mucociliary activity and ultrastructural abnormalities of regenerated sinus mucosa in rabbits. Laryngoscope 1994;104(12):1482–6.

[10] Orlandi RR, Kennedy DW. Surgical management of rhinosinusitis. Am J Med Sci 1998; 316(1):29–38.

[11] Orlandi RR, Lanza DC. Is nasal packing necessary following endoscopic sinus surgery? Laryngoscope 2004;114(9):1541–4.

[12] Perloff JR, Gannon FH, Bolger WE, et al. Bone involvement in sinusitis: an apparent pathway for the spread of disease. Laryngoscope 2000;110(12):2095–9.

[13] Stammberger H. Functional endoscopic sinus surgery. Philadelphia: B.C. Decker; 1991. p. 529.

[14] Hwang PH, McLaughlin RB, Lanza DC, et al. Endoscopic septoplasty: indications, technique, and results. Otolaryngol Head Neck Surg 1999;120(5):678–82.

[15] Orlandi RR, Kennedy DW. Revision endoscopic frontal sinus surgery. Otolaryngol Clin North Am 2001;34(1):77–90.

[16] Thornton R. Middle turbinate stabilization technique in endoscopic sinus surgery. Arch Otolaryngol Head Neck Surg 1996;122(8):869–72.

[17] Goldstein NA, Hebda PA, Klein EC, et al. Wound management of the airway mucosa: comparison with skin in a rabbit model. Int J Pediatr Otorhinolaryngol 1998;45:223–35.

[18] Lanza DC. Diagnosis of chronic rhinosinusitis. Ann Otol Rhinol Laryngol Suppl 2004;193: 10–4.

[19] Kuhn FA, Citardi MJ. Advances in postoperative care following functional endoscopic sinus surgery. Otolaryngol Clin North Am 1997;30(3):479–90.

[20] Chandra RK, Conley DB, Haines GK 3rd, et al. Long-term effects of FloSeal packing after endoscopic sinus surgery. Am J Rhinol 2005;19(3):240–3.

[21] Wallwork B, Coman W, Mackay-Sim A, et al. Effect of clarithromycin on nuclear factor-kappa B and transforming growth factor-beta in chronic rhinosinusitis. Laryngoscope 2004;114(2):286–90.

[22] Vaughan W. Audience response system in Nashville. Available at: http://american-rhinologic. org/.

[23] Kennedy DW. Prognostic factors, outcomes, and staging in ethmoid sinus surgery. Laryngoscope 1992;12(Suppl 57):1–18.

[24] Watelet JB, Claeys C, Van Cauwenberge P, et al. Predictive and monitoring value of matrix metalloproteinase-9 for healing quality after sinus surgery. Wound Repair Regen 2004;12(4): 412–8.

[25] Maccabee MS, Trune DR, Hwang PH. Paranasal sinus mucosal regeneration: the effect of topical retinoic acid. Am J Rhinol 2003;17(3):133–7.

[26] Chung JH, Cosenza MJ, Rahbar R, et al. Mitomycin C for the prevention of adhesion formation after endoscopic sinus surgery: a randomized, controlled study. Otolaryngol Head Neck Surg 2002;126(5):468–74.

[27] Ingrams DR, Volk MS, Biesman BS, et al. Sinus surgery: does mitomycin C reduce stenosis? Laryngoscope 1998;108:883–6.

[28] Rahal A, Peloquin L, Ahmarani C. Mitomycin C in sinus surgery: preliminary results in a rabbit model. J Otolaryngol 2001;30:1–5.

[29] Anand VK, Tabaee A, Kacker A, et al. The role of mitomycin C in preventing synechia and stenosis after endoscopic sinus surgery. Am J Rhinol 2004;18(5):311–4.

[30] Li H, Liu Y, Shu XZ, et al. Synthesis and biological evaluation of a cross-linked hyaluronan-mitomycin C hydrogel. Biomacromolecules 2004;5:895–902.

[31] Cai S, Liu Y, Zheng Shu X, et al. Injectable glycosaminoglycan hydrogels for controlled release of human basic fibroblast growth factor. Biomaterials 2005;26(30):6054–67.

[32] Proctor M, Proctor K, Shu XZ, et al. Composition of hyaluronan affects wound healing in the rabbit maxillary sinus. Am J Rhinol 2005.

[33] Gilbert ME, Kirker KR, Gray SD, et al. Chondroitin sulfate hydrogel and wound healing in rabbit maxillary sinus mucosa. Laryngoscope 2004;114(8):1406–9.

ELSEVIER
SAUNDERS

Otolaryngol Clin N Am
39 (2006) 475–492

OTOLARYNGOLOGIC
CLINICS
OF NORTH AMERICA

Reducing Complications in Rhinoplasty

Daniel G. Becker, MD, FACS[a,b,*],
Samuel S. Becker, MD[b]

[a]Division of Facial Plastic Surgery, Department of Otolaryngology,
University of Pennsylvania Medical Center, Philadelphia, PA
[b]University of Virginia Medical Center, Charlottesville, VA

The nose plays a functional role in nasal breathing and an esthetic role because it represents the most prominent and central facial feature. That the nose has enormous psychological, emotional, social, and symbolic importance is indisputable [1]. Studies suggest that most rhinoplasty patients benefit psychologically from the operation [1]. Although rhinoplasty can be a satisfying procedure for the patient and the surgeon, the literature reports an incidence of postoperative rhinoplasty complications ranging from 8% to 15%. The rhinoplasty surgeon must take great care to minimize the incidence of functional and cosmetic complications [2–10].

Ultimately, success in rhinoplasty is based on well-developed judgment, wisdom, and accumulated knowledge and experience. Similar to most surgeries, rhinoplasty is a science and an art. Skill comes from experience and wisdom, combined with a measure of talent. The surgeon must have a detailed understanding of the multiple anatomic variants encountered. The surgeon also must have accumulated the appropriate surgical techniques and experience. Specifically, the surgeon must acquire knowledge of the surgical alternatives, and how healing forces affect the result. This skill set is acquired by careful follow-up of operated patients over time.

There is no "standard" rhinoplasty. Each operation is unique in that it must be tailored to the specific anatomic components involved and the desires of the patient. By developing a consistent, meticulous routine in which the patient's nose is analyzed with regard to its anatomic components and their complex interrelationships, the surgeon can best select the appropriate incisions, approaches, and techniques for the patient's nose.

* Corresponding author. Becker Nose and Sinus Center, LLC 400 Medical Center Drive, Suite B, Sewell, NJ 08080.
    E-mail address: drbecker@therhinoplastycenter.com (D.G. Becker).

0030-6665/06/$ - see front matter © 2006 Elsevier Inc. All rights reserved.
doi:10.1016/j.otc.2006.01.002
oto.theclinics.com

The authors' philosophy of rhinoplasty focuses on achieving two essential goals. The first is to make the patient happy. Hand in hand is the second goal—for this to be their only cosmetic nasal surgery. With these goals in mind, this article presents the authors' personal philosophy and approach to reducing complications in rhinoplasty.

Cosmetic rhinoplasty patients: esthetic nasal examination

When the patient arrives at the office, he or she is greeted and are asked to fill out a detailed history form. The patient is taken to the photography room by a nurse assistant, who takes digital photographs and escorts the patient to the examination room. The nurse downloads the photographs into the network computer.

Next, the surgeon meets the patient. The surgeon asks what the patient does not like about his or her nose and what he or she would like the surgeon to fix. After the patient has explained his or her goals, the surgeon reviews any prior medical records. After a review of the medical history, the surgeon performs an examination.

Detailed anatomic analysis of the nose is an essential initial step in achieving a successful surgical outcome. The author's approach to rhinoplasty analysis in a primary rhinoplasty is well described [9]. Box 1 presents a partial list of specific considerations.

Rhinoplasty analysis

A thorough physical examination and accurate preoperative analysis are crucial to achieving the desired long-term postoperative rhinoplasty result. Some degree of mental organization assists in the execution of the physical examination. *Visual examination* and *finger palpation* are equally important in the nasal evaluation. Throughout the evaluation, a *mental image* of the potential outcome and surgical limitations inherent in every individual case should be visualized. In effect, the potential rhinoplasty operation is rehearsed even as the physical examination proceeds [9,11].

Study of the standard preoperative photographic images for rhinoplasty (frontal, base, lateral, oblique) allows a systematic, detailed anatomic analysis that complements the physical examination process. This section focuses on analysis of the four standard rhinoplasty photographic views (frontal, base, lateral, oblique). Emphasis is placed on anatomic descriptions of structures and their relationships to other structures.

Analysis begins by examining all four views and making an assessment of the overall stature of the patient, the facial skin quality, and the symmetry of the face. The quality of the skin–soft tissue envelope—its thickness, its quality, its integrity, and its mobility in relation to the underlying nasal structures—must be determined because it plays a crucial role in dictating the limitations of what can and cannot be accomplished with esthetic nasal surgery [9–12].

Box 1. Nasal analysis

General

Skin quality: integrity, vascularity, mobility, skin thickness (thin, medium, or thick)

Identify primary concerns leading patient to seek rhinoplasty (eg, "big," "twisted," "large hump")

Frontal view

Twisted or straight: follow brow-tip esthetic lines

Width: narrow, wide, normal, "wide-narrow-wide"

Tip: deviated, bulbous, asymmetric, amorphous, other

Base view

Triangularity: good versus trapezoidal

Tip: deviated, wide, bulbous, bifid, asymmetric

Base: wide, narrow, or normal; inspect for caudal septal deflection

Columella: columellar-to-lobule ratio (normal is 2:1 ratio); status of medial crural footplates

Lateral view

Nasofrontal angle: shallow or deep

Nasal starting point: high or low

Dorsum: straight, concavity, or convexity—bony, bony-cartilaginous or cartilaginous (ie, is convexity primarily bony, cartilaginous, or both)

Nasal length: normal, short, long

Tip projection: normal, decreased, or increased

Alar-columellar relationship: normal or abnormal

Nasolabial angle: obtuse or acute

Oblique view

Does it add anything, or does it confirm the other views

There are many other points of analysis that can be made on each view, but these are some of the vital points of commentary.

After completing the general assessment, the most striking characteristics of the nose should be noted and highlighted. These are typically the characteristics that bring the patient for rhinoplasty, such as excessive size, deviation, or a dorsal hump. These primary patient concerns must be recognized, highlighted, and addressed above all else.

As the surgeon reviews each photographic image, the major esthetic and technical points are noted first. Next, subtleties in analysis are addressed. It is important to recognize the characteristics of greatest concern to the patient

and the more subtle findings. The patient may not notice these other subtle abnormalities if they are left unaddressed by the surgeon. Postoperatively, the
scrutinizing patient may notice and point out these abnormalities. Stepwise,
methodical analysis of the patient and the photographic views allows
a well-trained surgeon to identify significant anatomic and esthetic points.

Frontal view

On frontal view, the observant surgeon first notes nasal width, any deviation from the midline, and characteristics of the nasal tip. Nasal width can
be assessed in the upper, middle, and lower third of the nose. A saddle deformity of the bony or cartilaginous dorsum contributes to the appearance
of an overwide dorsum on frontal view, whereas a hump gives the impression of a narrow dorsum. Similarly, a low bony dorsum creates an illusion
of a relatively wide upper third of the nose and wide intercanthal distance or
pseudohypertelorism [12]. This appearance can be improved significantly by
augmenting the nasal dorsum. The width of the nasal base on frontal view
should approximate the intercanthal distance.

The contour of the curved esthetic lines that follow the eyebrows, traverse
the radix, and continue down along the lateral nasal dorsum to end at the
tip-defining points (*brow-tip esthetic lines*) should be followed. Any asymmetries, twists, or deviations should be noted. These brow-tip esthetic lines
should be smooth, unbroken, gently curved, and symmetric [9,11].

The nasal tip should be characterized on frontal view with regard to symmetry and definition. Concavity or other anatomic findings of the alar side-
wall are noted. Vertical and horizontal aspects of bulbosity should be
recognized when present. Bifidity of the nasal tip may be visible on this
view (but is typically best appreciated on base view). The gentle "gull-in-
flight" relationship of the nasal alae to the infratip lobule should be followed, and any asymmetry should be noted. Exaggeration of this curve
suggests alar retraction or a dependent infratip lobule. If the columella is
not visible ("hidden columella") on frontal view, this also may indicate a retracted columella. The vertical position and symmetry of the alar insertions
should be described on the frontal view.

Base view

On base view, special attention should be given to triangularity, symmetry, columella-to-lobule ratio, and width and insertion of the alar base.
The nasal base should be configured as an isosceles triangle with a gently
rounded apex at the nasal tip and subtle flaring of the alar sidewalls
[13–15]. Poor triangularity or trapezoidal configuration with broad domal
angles may suggest abnormal divergence of the intermediate crura. The
presence of asymmetry of the tip may be appreciated best on this view. Often, one can visualize the outline of the lower lateral cartilages beneath the
thin skin of the columella and alar rim, and asymmetries or buckling can be

noted. Overlong or short medial crura may be apparent; a wide columella and flaring of the medial crural footplate should be noted when present. One should look into the nasal vestibule to identify possible recurvature of the lateral aspect of the lower lateral cartilage (lateral crura), which occasionally contributes to nasal obstruction or correlates with an alar concavity seen on frontal view. This recurvature of the lateral crura can be accentuated with application of dome-binding sutures (eg, transdomal sutures) resulting in nasal airway obstruction. The caudal septum may be seen protruding into a nostril. Asymmetric nostrils or protruding medial crural footplates may be a clue of subtle caudal septal deviation or asymmetry. Asymmetric orientation of the nostril apices may indicate underlying abnormalities of the domal region of the lower lateral cartilages.

The width of the alar base should be noted, with normal width generally being within a vertical line dropped from the medial canthi. Variations in the appearance of width on the base view may be due to the variation in horizontal position of the alar insertions on the face or in the flare of the alar sidewalls. The alar sidewalls themselves are characterized with regard to thickness and flare. Alar base insertions are described by degree of recurvature, with straight insertions going directly into the face (ie, no nostril sill), and extremely recurved alae inserting directly into the columella [13–15].

Lateral view

The lateral view offers important information on tip projection; nasal length; dorsal profile or contour, including the tip-supratip relationship; and alar-columellar relationship. The nasal tip ideally should project strongly from the face and lead gracefully to the supratip dorsum, creating a modest supratip break. An identifiable, but not overly exaggerated, columellar double break typically marks the junction of the medial and intermediate crus. Nasal tip projection is assessed consistently using the method described by Goode [16,17]. If the length of a line drawn from the tip-defining point perpendicular to a tangent to the alar-facial junction is greater than 0.55 to 0.60 of the line drawn from the nasion to tip-defining point, the nose may be overprojected. When assessing tip projection, relationships between the nose and other esthetic facial features (eg, chin projection, forehead contour, ethnic background) must be considered.

Nasal length is complicated to define. The objective definition of nasal length is the vertical distance from the nasion to the tip-defining point, and this measurement is compared with the other horizontal thirds of the face and the overall stature of the patient to determine if the nose is of appropriate length. The factors contributing to the appearance of nasal length are significantly more complex, however. The nose can be considered to have three lengths, with nasion to tip being the central length and nasion to alar margin being the lateral lengths. A short or long lateral length may reflect a retracted or hooded ala, whereas a short or long central length may reflect an obtuse or acute nasolabial (columellar-labial) angle. A deep nasofrontal angle contributes to the illusion of a short nose, and a shallow nasofrontal angle adds apparent length to the nose [18].

The nature of the columellar-labial confluence and columellar-lobular angle (double break) also must be assessed. Webbing or tenting of the columellar-labial confluence should be noted. An overly obtuse columellar-labial angle or an exaggerated double break makes the nose appear short, whereas the converse (acute columellar-labial angle or absent double break) adds apparent length. A posteriorly inclining lip or deficiency of the premaxilla may confound accurate measurement of the columellar-labial angle. Also, the relationship of the nose to other facial structures influences nasal length; a flat forehead gives the illusion of increased nasal length [18].

One should be familiar with the esthetic angles applied in facial analysis as general guidelines for standards of facial esthetics and facial harmony. The Powell and Humphries esthetic triangle (nasofacial, nasofrontal, nasomental, and mentocervical angles) and the nasolabial angle or confluence are a few of the more commonly cited measurements.

Assessment of the dorsal contour should identify any concavity, convexity, or irregularity. A high dorsum with a slight concavity at the rhinion generally is considered the esthetic ideal in the nose of a white woman. A high dorsum that is straight or with a small hump is ideal in a white man. Other notable components of the dorsum include the nasal starting point, which ideally is positioned at the level of the superior palpebral fold, and the tip-supratip relationship as previously mentioned.

The ala is analyzed in detail on the lateral view. Insertion of the ala on the face 2 to 3 mm above the columella in the horizontal plane as described by Crumley and Lanser [13] is judged to be normal. The contour of the alar rim in profile ideally approximates a "lazy S" shape—one should note if this is normal, exaggerated, or straight. The size of the alar lobule is classified as small, normal, or large. The alar-columellar relationship should be described precisely. The range of normal columellar show generally is considered to be 2 to 4 mm. The complexities of the alar-columellar relationship were categorized by Gunter et al [19], who identified abnormal positioning of the ala and the columella in relationship to a line drawn through the long axis of the nostril. All patients have a hanging, normal, or retracted ala and a hanging, normal, or retracted columella. The alar-columellar relationship comprises nine possible anatomic combinations.

On lateral view, the long axis of the nostril should rise at approximately 10° to 30° from a plane horizontal to the Frankfurt plane. This is a reliable determinant of the need for operative rotation of the nasal tip [12].

Oblique view

Although it offers the least amount of objective data, the oblique view is an important esthetic view because the nose is most often seen at oblique angles.

Several aspects of nasal contour are highlighted on this view and should be assessed. The brow-tip esthetic lines and the soft tissue facets are especially prominent and should be assessed carefully because irregularities may be highlighted on this view. Abnormalities of the lateral aspect of the nasal bones, nasal length, dorsal height, and tip projection also may be highlighted on the oblique view.

Functional nasal examination

Anterior rhinoscopy is undertaken and may identify abnormalities, such as deviated septum, inferior turbinate hypertrophy, synechiae or scar bands, septal perforation, and other abnormalities. Examination also includes nasal endoscopy when there is a complaint of nasal obstruction [20,21]. If indicated, a sinus CT scan also may be obtained.

Pownell et al [20] described diagnostic nasal endoscopy in the plastic surgical literature. They trace the historical development of nasal endoscopy, explain its rationale, review anatomic and diagnostic issues including the differential diagnosis of nasal obstruction, and describe the selection of equipment and correct application of technique, emphasizing the potential for advanced diagnostic potential.

Levine [21] reported that 39% of patients with a complaint of nasal obstruction had findings on endoscopic examination that were not identified with traditional rhinoscopy. Many of Levine's patients had seen other physicians for this problem and had not received appropriate treatment.

In patients seeking cosmetic nasal surgery who also had nasal obstruction, Becker et al [22,23] described how nasal endoscopy allowed the diagnosis of additional pathology not seen on anterior rhinoscopy, including obstructing adenoids, enlarged middle turbinates with concha bullosa, choanal stenosis, nasal polyps, and chronic sinusitis. In their series, additional surgical therapy was undertaken in 28 of 96 rhinoplasty patients as a result of findings on endoscopic examination. Thirteen patients had endoscopic sinus surgery. Nine patients had a concha bullosa requiring partial middle turbinectomy. Three patients—all revision surgeries—had persisting posterior septal deviation requiring endoscopic septoplasty. Two patients underwent adenoidectomy. One patient required repair of choanal stenosis. Static and dynamic nasal valve collapse occasionally is encountered in primary rhinoplasty patients [24]. In Becker et al's report [24], only 2 of 21 patients with nasal valve collapse reported no past history of rhinoplasty.

Discussion with patient

If, after careful examination, the patient's goals seem to be reasonable and realistic to this point, the surgeon tells the patient so. The surgeon explains technical details of the surgical plan to the patient. All rhinoplasty surgeons have complications. The literature reports complication rates of 8% to 15% [2–9]. Complications can occur despite surgery that has been well performed technically. The risk of complications is explained forthrightly to the patient. It is explained that, should a complication occur, it is generally correctible to some degree. The patient is informed that occasionally no improvement is possible.

Computer imaging

As part of the office consultation, computer imaging can be done. In the senior author's practice, the office computer network provides for imaging in each examination room. The patient's photos are uploaded onto the computer screen in the examination room, and computer imaging is undertaken.

The senior author explains to the patient that computer imaging is just a "video game"—that it is a way to communicate a shared surgical goal. This is *not* an "after" picture, it is *not* a guarantee, and it should *not* be taken to offer the slightest implication of a guarantee. It is simply a way to communicate the shared surgical goal. The senior author does not provide the patient with printouts of the computer imaging. The senior author explains to the patient that the preoperative photo and shared surgical goal photo routinely are printed out and taped to the wall in the operating room during surgery so that the pictures can be referred to as surgery progresses.

Typically, the surgeon and patient are able to reach a shared surgical goal. If so, the surgeon should reiterate his or her impression that the goals are reasonable and realistic. Technical details are discussed further. The potential benefits and potential risks of surgery are reviewed. After the surgeon and patient have concluded their discussion, the patient should be introduced to the office manager to discuss logistical and financial details.

Patient education

In the senior author's experience, the rhinoplasty patient researches the subject exhaustively. Many rhinoplasty patients avail themselves of the tremendous amount of educational material on the Internet. They are interested in learning about the procedure in general and are interested in preoperative and postoperative photographic images by their potential surgeon.

The best patient is a well-informed patient. In an effort to provide detailed information to individuals researching this subject, the senior author created two websites, www.TheRhinoplastyCenter.com and www.RevisionRhinoplasty.com. In addition to the requisite logistical information, considerable effort has been placed in providing a detailed educational tutorial at these websites. Consequently, the senior author has found that the patients he sees in the office already know "what is wrong" with their nose and already are reasonably well versed in the author's approach and philosophy.

Technical overview of potential complications

The nationally reported revision rate for primary rhinoplasty ranges from 8% to 15% [2–9]. Sadly, there will likely never be a shortage of patients requiring revision rhinoplasty. Experienced surgeons consistently achieve a high level of satisfaction among their patients. Still, complications can occur despite technically well-performed surgery. All surgeons have complications (Box 2).

Having the opportunity in practice to examine numerous revision rhinoplasty patients from across the United States and around the world, the senior author has observed a wide range of problems. The senior author has selected problems encountered in revision practice that warrant highlighting because they are problems encountered frequently or because they illustrate specific surgical techniques that may be particularly useful in the surgeon's armamentarium.

Specific problems to avoid

Overresection of lateral crura

Overresection of the lateral crus is perhaps the most common problem seen in a revision rhinoplasty practice [6,10,24–27]. Overresection of the lateral crus leads to the predictable changes of alar retraction, pinching, bossae, and tip asymmetry (Fig. 1). Excision of vestibular mucosa in primary rhinoplasty also may contribute to scar contracture with alar retraction. A conservative approach to cephalic resection is warranted in rhinoplasty.

In many revision cases, the amount of lateral crus that remained seemed ample; that is, it fell within the "guideline" of 6 to 9 mm that typically is cited. In these cases, the scar contracture secondary to healing apparently overpowered the remnant cartilage. If the tip cartilages are soft and weak, and if the scar contracture is profound, undesirable changes can occur.

In some cases, this situation can be anticipated. An anatomic study of the alar base recognized that in a normal patient population, 20% of patients had a thin alar rim. This anatomic variation must be recognized, and cephalic resection probably should be avoided or minimized in these patients to minimize the risk of alar retraction or external nasal valve collapse [25]. These changes are not always predictable, however, and are not always avoidable.

Understanding that the healing forces are not completely predictable, it is important to take a conservative approach when undertaking cephalic resection. Risk cannot be eliminated, but can be reduced in this manner.

Alar batten grafts are the first-line treatment of alar retraction and nasal valve collapse (Fig. 2) [10,24,26]. Batten grafts have been well described in the literature. Alar retraction may be treated by cartilage batten grafts in less severe cases (1–2 mm) [9].

Auricular composite grafts commonly are used in more severe cases (Fig. 3) [27]. The skin and cartilage of the anterolateral surface, just inferior

---

Box 2. Complications of rhinoplasty

Bossae
Bossae are caused by a knuckling of lower lateral cartilage at the nasal tip owing to contractural healing forces acting on weakened cartilages. Patients with thin skin, strong cartilages, and nasal tip bifidity are especially at risk. Excessive resection of lateral crus and failure to eliminate excessive interdomal width may play some role in bossae formation.

Pollybeak
Pollybeak refers to postoperative fullness of the supratip, with an abnormal tip-supratip relationship. It has several etiologies, including failure to maintain adequate tip support (postoperative loss of tip projection), inadequate cartilaginous hump (anterior septal angle) removal, or supratip dead space/scar formation.
Treatment depends on anatomic cause. If the cartilaginous hump was underresected, one should resect additional dorsal septum. Also, one must ensure adequate tip support. Maneuvers such as placement of a columellar strut may be beneficial. If the bony hump was overresected, one should consider a graft to augment the bony dorsum. If a pollybeak is from excessive scar formation, triamcinolone (Kenalog) injection or skin taping should be considered in the early postoperative period, before any consideration of surgical revision.

Inverted V deformity
Inadequate support of the upper lateral cartilages after dorsal hump removal can lead to inferomedial collapse of the upper lateral cartilages and an inverted V deformity. In this deformity, the caudal edge of the nasal bones is visible in broad relief, frequently owing to inadequate infracture of the nasal bones. When executing hump excision, it is helpful to preserve the underlying nasal mucoperichondrium (extramucosal dissection), which provides significant support to the upper lateral cartilages and helps decrease the risk of inferomedial collapse of the upper lateral cartilages after hump excision. When undertaking osteotomies after hump excision, appropriate infracture and narrowing of the bony vault must be achieved.

> ## Rocker deformity
> If osteotomies are taken too high, into the thick frontal bone, the superior aspect of the osteotomized nasal bone may project or "rock" laterally when the bone is infractured. This is a rocker deformity. A 2-mm osteotome may be employed percutaneously to create a more appropriate superior fracture line and correct the rocker deformity.
>
> ## Dorsal irregularities
> After creation of an "open roof" by hump removal, the bony margins should be smoothed with a rasp. Any bony fragments should be removed, ensuring that all obvious particles are removed from under the skin–soft tissue envelope. Failure to remove all fragments may lead to a visible or palpable dorsal irregularity.
>
> ## Nasal valve collapse
> The surgeon should recognize the existence of the internal and external nasal valve. The internal nasal valve is bounded by the caudal margin of the upper lateral cartilage, septum, and floor of the nose. The external nasal valve refers to the area delineated by the cutaneous and skeletal support of the mobile alar wall. Excessive narrowness in either of these locations may cause nasal obstruction. Weakness at either of these locations may result in collapse with the negative pressure of inspiration, resulting in nasal airway obstruction. Nasal valve collapse is seen most often as a sequela of overresection of lateral crura or middle vault collapse. Overaggressive resection of the lateral crura and the subsequent postoperative soft tissue contraction frequently lead to nasal valve compromise.

to the inferior crus, of the opposite ear (eg, left ala, right ear) provides the best donor site and the best contour. An incision several millimeters from the nostril rim is followed by careful dissection with freeing of adhesions, creating a defect and displacing the alar rim inferiorly. Volume and support must be restored to hold the nostril rim in position—this role is fulfilled by the composite graft. The fashioned composite graft is sutured carefully into place [27]. Typically, the senior author uses 5-0 chromic suture. A cotton ball or other light dressing is applied intranasally to apply light pressure for 1 to 3 days.

Minimizing nasal dorsum complications

Sharp osteotomes are essential to provide for a clean, precise bony hump excision. When the osteotome is dull, the chance of an asymmetric resection or overresection of the bony hump increases. Some surgeons have at least

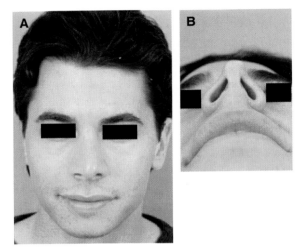

Fig. 1. Overresection of the nasal tip cartilages in this patient resulted in predictable, unfavorable changes. (Copyright © Daniel Becker, MD)

two sets of osteotomes and rotate them—one set is always out, being sharpened. Other surgeons sharpen their osteotomes manually, with a sharpening stone, during each case. Both approaches are effective.

An anatomic approach is preferable. Detailed anatomic nasal analysis should guide surgery. When undertaking a hump reduction, the surgeon

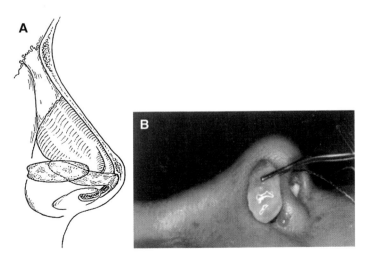

Fig. 2. Alar batten grafts may be placed via an external rhinoplasty approach or into a precise pocket made through an endonasal incision as shown here. This graft is nonanatomic and typically is placed caudal to the lateral crura, where there is maximal collapse of the lateral nasal wall and supra-alar pinching. For maximal support, the alar batten graft should extend over the bone of the piriform aperture. (Copyright © Daniel Becker, MD)

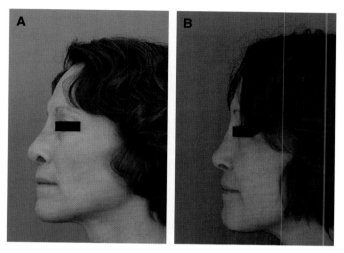

Fig. 3. Composite grafts are useful in the treatment of severe alar retraction. (Copyright © Daniel Becker, MD)

should examine the excised tissue, assessing its symmetry, and whether it was the desired excision. If the bony dorsum is rasped, this would not be possible (Fig. 4). Similar anatomic examination of the remaining cartilaginous and bony nasal dorsum also must be undertaken. It is expected that additional, calibrated refinement would be needed and should be undertaken with dogmatic adherence to the anatomic examination. Preoperative markings on the skin may be helpful to some surgeons for hump reduction and for osteotomies. Persistent irregularities of the bony dorsum may be

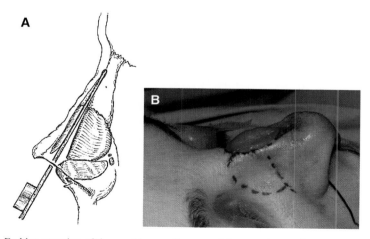

Fig. 4. En bloc resection of the nasal hump allows careful anatomic examination as the surgeon assesses the need for additional, calibrated refinements of the nasal dorsum. (Copyright © Daniel Becker, MD)

addressed by rasping. The powered rasp is preferable to manual rasping in this situation (Fig. 5) [28,29].

Pollybeak

Pollybeak refers to a specific problem of the nasal dorsum—postoperative fullness of the supratip region, with an abnormal tip-supratip relationship. This problem may have several causes, including failure to maintain adequate tip support (postoperative loss of tip projection), inadequate cartilaginous hump (anterior septal angle) removal, or supratip dead space or scar formation. Treatment of the pollybeak deformity depends on the anatomic cause [30]. The best treatment is avoidance. If the cartilaginous hump was underresected at the anterior septal angle, however, the revision surgeon should resect additional dorsal septum. Adequate tip support must be ensured; maneuvers such as placement of a columellar strut may be beneficial. If the bony hump was overresected, a graft to augment the bony dorsum may be beneficial. If a pollybeak is from excessive scar formation, triamcinolone (Kenalog) injection or skin taping in the early postoperative period should be undertaken before any consideration of surgical revision.

Overresection and saddle nose

Saddle nose refers to the appearance of the nose after loss of support of the nasal vault with subsequent collapse (Fig. 6). This deformity has been described after overresection of the septum, with failure to preserve an adequate L-strut. A minimum of 15 mm of cartilage is recommended as a rule of thumb—if a dorsal hump resection also is planned, this must be accounted for in planning adequate L-strut for nasal support. Other causes of saddle nose deformity include septal hematoma, septal abscess, and severe nasal trauma. Excessive dorsal hump resection also leads to saddle-nose deformity.

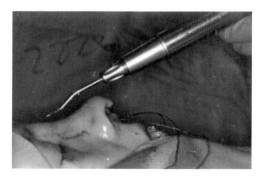

Fig. 5. The powered rasp (Linvatec-Hall Surgical, Largo, FL) oscillates at speeds of 15,000 rpm with minimal back-and-forth excursion of only several millimeters. The senior author finds the powered rasp more precise and preferable to manual rasping. (Copyright © Daniel Becker, MD)

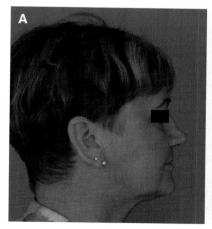 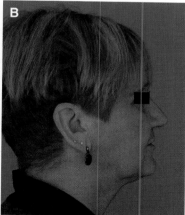

Fig. 6. Precise pocket, triple-layer cartilage onlay grafting effectively treated this patient's saddle-nose deformity. (Copyright © Daniel Becker, MD)

Onlay grafting can camouflage and correct mild and moderate saddle deformities effectively (Fig. 6). Single or multiple layers of septal cartilage or auricular cartilage commonly are used effectively [31,32]. Severe saddle-nose deformity may require major reconstruction with cantilevered cartilage or bone grafts [33,34].

Alloplasts

The senior author's experience with alloplasts has been to remove them. The author has removed alloplasts because they cause pain, because they caused an unacceptable cosmetic result, because they became infected, and because of extrusion into the nose and through the skin. There is disagreement among rhinoplasty surgeons regarding the use of alloplasts. The nose fulfills few of the requirements for use of alloplastic materials. If the alloplast extrudes through the skin, the skin–soft tissue envelope is permanently and irreparably damaged. The senior author discourages the use of alloplasts in primary and revision rhinoplasty.

Inverted V–middle vault collapse

In inverted V–middle vault collapse deformity, the caudal edge of the nasal bones are visible in broad relief. Inadequate support of the upper lateral cartilages after dorsal hump removal can lead to inferomedial collapse of the upper lateral cartilages and an inverted V deformity [35]. Inadequate infracture of the nasal bones is another significant cause of inverted V deformity. The anatomic cause of inverted V deformity must be recognized. Osteotomies with infracture of the nasal bones, spreader grafts, or both should be performed when appropriate.

Twisted nose—newly or persistently twisted

Persisting deviation after rhinoplasty may occur at the upper third, middle third, or tip of the nose or may occur postoperatively in a previously straight nose. Preoperative anatomic diagnosis is a crucial component of successful treatment. Persisting deviation of the nasal bones may occur because of greenstick fractures or other problems with osteotomies [36,37]. Inherent deviations in the cartilage of the middle nasal vault may prove especially challenging [37]. Also, hump removal may uncover asymmetries that result in postoperative deviation where none existed previously. Tip asymmetry may be overlooked preoperatively, or it may due to asymmetric excision of lateral crura, asymmetric placement of a columellar strut, placement of an overlong columellar strut, or other causes. Numerous surgical maneuvers are available to address the deviated nose [36,37].

Skin–soft tissue envelope

In the unoperated nose, the skin–soft tissue envelope has well-defined tissue planes in which avascular dissection may be undertaken. Vascular supply and lymphatics are found superficial to the nasal musculature [38,39]. Dissection in the proper tissue planes (areolar tissue plane, ie, submusculoaponeurotic) preserves nasal blood supply and minimizes postoperative edema. Operating in the more superficial planes not only leads to a bloody surgical field, but also risks damage to the vascular supply with potential damage to the skin. When the skin–soft tissue envelope is damaged, it can never be restored fully. The damaged skin creates an esthetically displeasing appearance [38,39].

Summary

The dedicated rhinoplasty surgeon continues to acquire throughout his or her career an increasingly detailed understanding of the anatomy and the problems that occur related to rhinoplasty and a growing armamentarium of techniques to achieve improvement or correction. This article outlines the authors' approach and discusses selected technical problems and approaches to reducing their occurrence. Focusing on the two essential goals—making the patient happy and making this the patient's only nasal surgery—primary rhinoplasty can be a uniquely rewarding experience for the patient and the surgeon.

References

[1] Goin JM, Goin MK. Changing the body—psychological effects of plastic surgery. Baltimore: Williams & Wilkins; 1981.
[2] Kamer FM, Pieper PG. Revision rhinoplasty. In: Bailey B, editor. Head and neck surgery otolaryngology. Philadelphia: Lippincott; 1998. p. 2291–302.

[3] Rees TD. Postoperative considerations and complications. In: Rees TD, editor. Aesthetic plastic surgery. Philadelphia: Saunders; 1980.

[4] McKinney P, Cook JQ. A critical evaluation of 200 rhinoplasties. Ann Plast Surg 1981; 7:357.

[5] Thomas JR, Tardy ME. Complications of rhinoplasty. Ear Nose Throat J 1986;65:19–34.

[6] Tardy ME, Cheng EY, Jernstrom V. Misadventures in nasal tip surgery. Otolaryngol Clin North Am 1987;20:797–823.

[7] Simons RL, Gallo JF. Rhinoplasty complications. Facial Plast Surg Clin N Am 1994;2: 521–9.

[8] Becker DG. Complications in rhinoplasty. In: Papel I, editor. Facial plastic and reconstructive surgery. 2nd edition. New York: Theime; 2002.

[9] Tardy ME. Rhinoplasty: the art and the science. Philadelphia: Saunders; 1997.

[10] Toriumi DM, Becker DG. Rhinoplasty dissection manual. Philadelphia: Lippincott Williams & Wilkins; 1999.

[11] Tardy ME, Brown R. Surgical anatomy of the nose. New York: Raven Press; 1990.

[12] Johnson CM, Toriumi DM. Open structure rhinoplasty. Philadelphia: Saunders; 1990.

[13] Crumley RL, Lanser M. Quantitative analysis of nasal tip projection. Laryngoscope 1998; 98:202–8.

[14] Tardy ME, Patt BS, Walter MA. Alar reduction and sculpture: anatomic concepts. Facial Plast Surg 1993;9:295–305.

[15] Becker DG, Weinberger MS, Greene BA, Tardy ME. Clinical study of alar anatomy and surgery of the alar base. Arch Otolaryngol Head Neck Surg 123:789–95.

[16] Tardy ME, Walter MA, Patt BS. The overprojecting nose: anatomic component analysis and repair. Facial Plast Surg 1993;9:306–16.

[17] Ridley MB. Aesthetic facial proportions. In: Papel I, Nachlas N, editors. Facial plastic and reconstructive surgery. Philadelphia: Mosby-Year Book; 1992. p. 99–109.

[18] Tardy ME, Becker DG, Weinberger MS. Illusions in rhinoplasty. Facial Plast Surg 1995;11: 117–38.

[19] Gunter JP, Rohrich RJ, Friedman RM. Classification and correction of alar-columellar discrepancies in rhinoplasty. Plast Reconstr Surg 1996;97:643–8.

[20] Pownell PH, Minoli JJ, Rohrich RJ. Diagnostic nasal endoscopy. Plast Reconstr Surg 1997; 99:1451–8.

[21] Levine HL. The office diagnosis of nasal and sinus disorders using rigid nasal endoscopy. Otolaryngol Head Neck Surg 1990;102:370.

[22] Becker DG. Septoplasty and turbinate surgery. Aesthetic Surg J 2003;23:393–403.

[23] Lanfranchi PV, Steiger J, Sparano A, et al. Diagnostic and surgical endoscopy in functional septorhinoplasty. Facial Plast Surg 2004;20:207–15.

[24] Becker DG, Becker SS. Alar batten grafts for treatment of nasal valve collapse. Journal of the Long-Term Effects of Surgical Implants 2003;13:259–69.

[25] Becker DG, Weinberger MS, Greene BA, Tardy ME. Clinical study of alar anatomy and surgery of the alar base. Arch Otolaryngol Head Neck Surg 1999;123:789–95.

[26] Toriumi DM, Josen J, Weinberger MS, Tardy ME. Use of alar batten grafts for correction of nasal valve collapse. Arch Otol Head Neck Surg 1997;123:802–8.

[27] Tardy ME, Toriumi DM. Alar retraction: composite graft correction. Facial Plast Surg 1989;6:101–7.

[28] Becker DG, Park SS, Toriumi DM. Powered instrumentation for rhinoplasty and septoplasty. Otolaryngol Clin North Am 1999;32:683–93.

[29] Becker DG, Toriumi DM, Gross CW, Tardy ME. Powered instrumentation for dorsal nasal reduction. Facial Plast Surg 1997;13:291–7.

[30] Tardy ME, Kron TK, Younger RY, Key M. The cartilaginous pollybeak: etiology, prevention, and treatment. Facial Plast Surg 1989;6:113–20.

[31] Tardy ME, Schwartz M, Parras G. Saddle nose deformity: autogenous graft repair. Facial Plast Surg 1989;6:121–34.

[32] Gunter JP, Rohrich RJ. Augmentation rhinoplasty: dorsal onlay grafting using shaped autogenous septal cartilage. Plast Reconstr Surg 1990;86:39–45.
[33] Daniel RK. Rhinoplasty and rib grafts: evolving a flexible operative technique. Plast Reconstr Surg 1992;94:597–611.
[34] Murakami CS, Cook TA, Guida RA. Nasal reconstruction with articulated irradiated rib
cartilage. Arch Otolaryngol Head Neck Surg 1991;117:327–30.
[35] Toriumi DM. Management of the middle nasal vault. Oper Tech Plast Reconst Surg 1995;2:
16–30.
[36] Larrabee WF Jr. Open rhinoplasty and the upper third of the nose. Facial Plast Surg Clin N
Am 1993;1:23–38.
[37] Toriumi DM, Ries WR. Innovative surgical management of the crooked nose. Facial Plast
Surg Clin N Am 1993;1:63–78.
[38] Rettinger G, Zenkel M. Skin and soft tissue complications. Facial Plast Surg 1997;13:51–9.
[39] Toriumi DM, Mueller RA, Grosch T, et al. Vascular anatomy of the nose and the external
rhinoplasty approach. Arch Otol Head Neck Surg 1996;122:24–34.

ELSEVIER
SAUNDERS

Otolaryngol Clin N Am
39 (2006) 493–501

OTOLARYNGOLOGIC
CLINICS
OF NORTH AMERICA

Endonasal Laser Surgery: An Update

Howard L. Levine, MD[a,b,c,]*

[a]*Cleveland Nasal-Sinus & Sleep Center, 5555 Transportation Blvd., Suite C, Cleveland, OH 44125, USA*
[b]*Marymount Outpatient Care Center, Marymount Hospital, Garfield Heights, OH, USA*
[c]*The Cleveland Clinic Head and Neck Institute, Cleveland, OH, USA*

Although surgical lasers were introduced more than 30 years ago, their use and popularity in nasal and sinus disease have been limited. Even so, there are many practitioners who find the laser a valuable surgical tool for nasal and sinus disease, either alone or in combination with other treatment modalities [1–6]. Those who do not use lasers probably do not because of a lack of skill, knowledge, or understanding of the role and availability of the technology. This article reviews the history and current role of lasers in nasal and sinus surgery.

Types of lasers typically used for endonasal surgery

Carbon dioxide laser

The carbon dioxide laser is delivered generally through an articulated arm using an argon-beam-aiming laser for accuracy. The laser can be used with microscope or appropriate hand pieces. The laser energy does not pass through glass, making typical eyeglasses safe. The carbon dioxide laser has a wavelength of 10.6 nanometers (nm). Its wavelength permits excellent absorption by water, which is the major component of most cells. There is very little damage to adjacent tissue. Generally, it can coagulate blood vessels up to 0.5 mm in diameter, thereby permitting reasonable hemostasis in most surgical situations. There is a shallow depth of penetration due to rapid heat loss caused by the evaporation of intracellular water. The carbon dioxide laser has excellent soft tissue interaction and good hemostasis for small to midsized capillaries.

---

* Cleveland Nasal-Sinus & Sleep Center, 5555 Transportation Blvd., Suite C, Cleveland, OH 44125, USA.
E-mail address: HLevine@ClevelandNasalSinus.com

Disadvantages include the smoke produced and the poor bone interaction [7,8]. The carbon dioxide laser is difficult to use within the nose and sinuses because there are no flexible fibers. The laser energy must be directed straight ahead or angled off front-faced mirrors. There is some concern about using the carbon dioxide laser in the sinuses because no reliable studies exist that demonstrate the effect of the laser on the bone underlying the sinus mucosa. Some of the bony sinus walls are thin and the heat of the laser could potentially damage the thin bone or underlying tissue.

KTP laser

The potassium titanyl phosphate (KTP) laser has a wavelength of 532 nm and is similar to an argon laser. It is delivered through a flexible fiber of 0.6 nm. Flexible fibers can be directed through angled suctions to reach most areas of the nasal cavity and sinuses [2,9]. Like the argon laser, it is absorbed selectively by pigmented tissue and poorly by pale tissue. It has a slightly less precise cutting ability than the carbon dioxide laser and better coagulating effect than the neodymium YAG laser. The KTP laser has been used for many types of sinus and nasal pathology [10]. Wound healing is quick with minimal adjacent tissue damage [11].

Holmium YAG laser

The holmium:yttrium-aluminum-garnet (YAG) laser is a solid-state laser of 2.1 nm wavelength. It is delivered through a pulsed operating system in an infrared spectrum. It can be coupled with various instruments for use in the nose and sinuses [12,13]. The YAG laser's wavelength and energy give it the ability to penetrate and obliterate bone [14]. Its wavelength is not as well absorbed by water as that of the carbon dioxide laser so tissue penetration is generally greater. However, penetration is not as deep as that of the neodymium YAG laser, making it a safer laser to use when working in the paranasal sinuses [15]. It has been used in orthopedic surgery and ophthalmology for darcryocystorhinostomy (DCR) [5,6].

Types of pathology managed and results

Nasal turbinates

Vasomotor rhinitis and allergic rhinitis are usually managed medically with oral decongestants, steroid nasal sprays, or in acute and short-term usage, topical nasal decongestants. In spite of adequate medical management, some patients either do not wish to use the medications, cannot tolerate them, or find them ineffective. For these patients, laser turbinate reduction, either by coagulating to create scar, reduce obstruction, and decrease drainage [16–22], or as a partial turbinate removal, may provide relief [23–25].

Mittleman [26], Elwany and colleagues [27,28], and Mladina and colleagues [29] used the carbon dioxide laser to perform partial turbinectomy for obstructive nasal symptoms of perennial rhinitis. Mittleman vaporized the anterior half of the inferior turbinate and achieved excellent results.

Kawamura and colleagues and Fukutake [30,31] describe the use of the carbon dioxide laser for allergic rhinitis. The inferior turbinates of 389 subjects with perennial allergic rhinitis were vaporized by a defocused carbon dioxide laser. They used the laser at 12 watts and 0.1 seconds at weekly intervals for 5 weeks. One month after surgery, 78% of the subjects had excellent or good results, whereas 21% professed no improvement. Seventy-two of the 389 subjects were followed for over 2 years, and 61 of the 72 had excellent or good results. Twenty-seven of the 72 subjects needed repeat vaporization. In a previous report, Fukutake and colleagues [31,32] described histologic studies that showed a layer of scar tissue forming beneath the submucosa. It is thought that the scar tissue prevents the turbinate from expanding when stimulated by external irritants.

The carbon dioxide laser is also useful and effective for nasal obstruction. Lagerholm and colleagues [16] describe its long-term effectiveness. Twenty-four to 36 months after treatment, three quarters of the subjects reported a marked decrease in nasal obstruction, as well as a reduced frequency in nasal and sinus infections.

A group of 1003 subjects who underwent KTP reduction of the turbinate has been followed for over 10 years by the author [2,10,33]. Eight hundred ninety-six of these subjects were available for follow-up. These subjects had had laser reduction performed under attended local anesthesia, or general anesthesia if the procedure was associated with a septoplasty. Septoplasty was performed in 645 (72%) of the 896 cases. The laser was used at 8 watts and was continuous in order to "cross-hatch" the anterior two thirds of the inferior turbinate. This allowed the nasal mucosa to regenerate, preserving a "normal" surface while creating a layer of scar tissue in the submucosa. Four hundred ninety-eight (55.5%) of the 896 subjects had extensive improvement in breathing; 197 (22%) had moderate improvement; 113 (12.6%) had mild improvement; and 88 (9.8%) had no improvement. Three hundred eighty-nine (43.4%) of the subjects had extensive reduction in their nasal drainage; 269 (30.0%) had moderate reduction; 132 (14.7%) had mild reduction; and 106 (11.8%) had no change in their nasal drainage. No subject reported being worse.

Because laser turbinate reduction is performed on the surface of the turbinate, there is some swelling, crusting and atrophy, but it is minimal [11,34]. If the laser turbinate reduction is performed in combination with endoscopic sinus surgery, the swelling and crusting may make immediate postoperative care difficult. This should be kept in mind when choosing a method to manage turbinate dysfunction.

Healing is rapid and morbidity low. The laser improves the airway and reduces secretions in most instances.

Endoscopic sinus surgery

Lasers have been tried in many different areas of endoscopic sinus surgery. In some areas the laser is effective but in others it is cumbersome and tedious. It has been used to create nasal antral windows in a controlled and minimally invasive manner, in an attempt to minimize scar tissue and improve window patency [35].

Metson [36] reports using the holmium:YAG (Ho:YAG) laser for endoscopic sinus surgery. He found the bone removal to be effective and equivalent to conventional endoscopic sinus surgery. Both methods allow the relief of symptoms and disease. The laser was effective in the removal of the thicker dense bone. It also provided safe removal of the thin eggshell bone around the ethmoid and orbit.

Gerlinger and colleagues [9] and the author [10] have successfully used the KTP laser for endoscopic sinus surgery. It was possible to use the laser because the flexible fibers and angled hand pieces permitted access into most or all of the sinus areas (Fig. 1).

Dacryocystorhinostomy

Several methods have been used for dacryocystorhinostomy (DCR). The typical method employed has been the use of a drill for managing the lacrimal bone. Several lasers have been tried in an attempt to get through the bone and create a communication between the lacrimal sack and the ethmoid sinus (and subsequently the nasal cavity). The Ho:YAG laser has seemed to be the most effective for removal of this thicker bone [37–39]. Overall ostium patency has been over 80% [40].

Sinus and nasal polyps

Ohyama [41] has described the use of polyp removal with the laser. The author attempted to use the laser for the removal of polyps (personal unpublished work). The concept was to vaporize the interstitial fluid component of the polyp and shrink the polyps. Although this concept seemed to make sense, it was tedious and difficult. Attempts to remove the polyps by excising them along their roots were similarly tedious. Visualization was also difficult. (Other types of lasers and instrumentation that will be

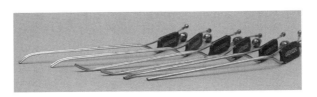

Fig. 1. Hand pieces that permit the use of flexible fibers.

developed in the future may make this approach technically and clinically feasible.)

Rhinologists have struggled with the management of patients with triad asthma, nasal polyposis, and aspirin sensitivity. After conventional removal of sinus and nasal polyps, the laser has been used to photocoagulate the bed in an attempt to create scar tissue and prevent recurrence. This was successful in 15 subjects who have been followed for about 10 to 16 years (personal unpublished work by author).

Choanal atresia

Choanal atresia can be membranous, bony or a combination of the two. The laser can provide assistance in the removal of the atretic tissue, when combined with either microscope or endoscope. The laser, coupled with nasal endoscopy or microscope, permits a one-stage repair with minimal tissue trauma [42–50]. The choice of the laser might depend on whether the tissue is bone or soft tissue.

Epistaxis

Typically, epistaxis is managed easily with chemical or electrical cautery. However, epistaxis from abnormal vascular malformations often can be managed most effectively with laser. The argon or KTP laser works best for this type of pathology. These entities may include hemangiomata [10,51], granulation tissue, prominent blood vessels, or hereditary hemorrhagic telangiectasia [52–54].

For vascular disorders, it is best to begin peripherally by photocoagulating the tissue around the lesion, and then work toward the center. This minimizes the bleeding.

Neoplasia

The laser is probably not the best way to manage most nasal and sinus neoplasms. There is no good data to substantiate effectiveness as a primary oncologic tool. However, for some neoplasia of the sinuses, it has been used as a reasonable adjunctive tool. It has been combined with conventional endoscopic sinus surgery to outline and theoretically seal the tissue between the neoplasm and normal tissue, preventing tumor spread and creating a more acceptable oncologic resection.

Inverted papilloma is the neoplasm resected most commonly with laser [10]. This permits the outline of the incision with minimal bleeding and then removal of the tumor. The laser has also been used to photocoagulate the base of the inverted papilloma in an attempt to obliterate cells with the potential for regrowth of the tumor [2,55,56].

The laser can be used in an adjunctive manner to remove osteomataby vaporizing the bone in a controlled manner [57].

Limitations of endonasal laser surgery

Cost

One of the limitations of using lasers as part of any type of surgery is cost effectiveness. Because most lasers are purchased by a surgery center or operating room, there must be some proven cost benefit. In addition, because there is no specific coding for reimbursement, the ability to acquire lasers for nasal and sinus surgery is limited. Some institutions have begun to rent lasers; this is a more cost-efficient means of having the technology availability.

Instrumentation

Lasers have several different wavelengths that improve their use for different types of tissues and have different efficiencies for surgical cutting or coagulation. However, one of the difficulties of laser use for nasal and sinus surgery is the inability to get into the various recesses and spaces of the nasal and sinus cavities. Flexible fibers inserted through angled hand pieces can be used easily with nasal endoscopes to work on almost all of the lateral walls of the nose and go into all of the various sinuses. These are light, easily handled, and have the additional benefit of suction to remove smoke from the operating field. Some lasers require special filters to protect the surgeon and operating room staff. Coupling these with nasal endoscopes can be cumbersome. Adding computer-guided surgical systems or irrigating devices to the endoscopes also makes the instrumentation heavy and difficult to manage.

Time consumption

The laser, while effective for many tissue types and pathologies, does seem to be time consuming because it is slow in its obliteration and vaporization of tissue.

The ideal rhinologic laser

The ideal rhinologic laser is probably not yet developed and in clinical use. Laryngeal lasers are used for removal of soft tissue; however, the rhinologic laser needs to ablate dense bone, remove soft tissue, and coagulate a dense vascular bed. It must do this in an efficient way. It must have flexible fibers and a delivery system that reaches the recesses and spaces of the nose and sinuses. It must have a depth of penetration sufficient to remove tissue while preserving and protecting the underlying important structures surrounding the sinuses.

References

[1] Kaluskar SK. Laser surgery in the management of sinonasal disease. Hosp Med 2004;65(8):
    476–80.

[2] Levine HL. Endoscopy and the KTP/532 laser for nasal sinus disease. Ann Otol Rhinol Laryngol 1989;98(1 Pt 1):46–51.

[3] Pothman R, Yeh HL. The effects of treatment with antibiotics, laser and acupuncture upon chronic maxillary sinusitis in children. Am J Chin Med 1982;10(1–4):55–8.

[4] Rathfoot CJ, Duncavage J, Shapshay SM. Laser use in the paranasal sinuses. Otolaryngol Clin North Am 1996;29(6):943–8.

[5] Shapshay SM, Rebeiz EE, Bohigian RK, et al. Holmium: yttrium aluminum garnet laser-assisted endoscopic sinus surgery: laboratory experience. Laryngoscope 1991;101(2):142–9.

[6] Shapshay SM, Rebeiz EE, Pankratov MM. Holmium:yttrium aluminum garnet laser-assisted endoscopic sinus surgery: clinical experience. Laryngoscope 1992;102(10):1177–80.

[7] Gonzalez C, van de Merwe WP, Smith M, et al. Comparison of the erbium-yttrium aluminum garnet and carbon dioxide lasers for in vitro bone and cartilage ablation. Laryngoscope 1990;100(1):14–7.

[8] Stasche N, Hormann K, Christ M, et al. Carbon dioxide laser delivery systems in functional paranasal sinus surgery. Adv Otorhinolaryngol 1995;49:114–7.

[9] Gerlinger I, Lujber L, Jarai T, et al. KTP-532 laser-assisted endoscopic nasal sinus surgery. Clin Otolaryngol 2003;28(2):67–71.

[10] Levine HL. Lasers in endonasal surgery. Otolaryngol Clin North Am 1997;30(3):451–5.

[11] Kass EG, Massaro BM, Komorowski RA, et al. Wound healing of KTP and argon laser lesions in the canine nasal cavity. Otolaryngol Head Neck Surg 1993;108(3):283–92.

[12] Feyh J. Endoscopic surgery of the nose and paranasal sinuses with the aid of the holmium: YAG laser. Adv Otorhinolaryngol 1995;49:122–4.

[13] Gleich LL, Rebeiz EE, Pankratov MM, et al. The holmium:YAG laser-assisted otolaryngologic procedures. Arch Otolaryngol Head Neck Surg 1995;121(10):1162–6.

[14] Stein E, Sedlacek T, Fabian RL, et al. Acute and chronic effects of bone ablation with a pulsed holmium laser. Lasers Surg Med 1990;10(4):384–8.

[15] von Glass W, Hauerstein T. Wound healing in the nose and paranasal sinuses after irradiation with the argon laser. An experimental study in animals. Arch Otorhinolaryngol 1988; 245(1):36–41.

[16] Lagerholm S, Harsten G, Emgard P, et al. Laser-turbinectomy: long-term results. J Laryngol Otol 1999;113(6):529–31.

[17] Wolfson S, Wolfson LR, Kaplan I. CO2 laser inferior turbinectomy: a new surgical approach. J Clin Laser Med Surg 1996;14(2):81–3.

[18] Takeno S, Osada R, Ishino T, et al. Laser surgery of the inferior turbinate for allergic rhinitis with seasonal exacerbation: an acoustic rhinometry study. Ann Otol Rhinol Laryngol 2003; 112(5):455–60.

[19] Passali D, Lauriello M, Anselmi M, et al. Treatment of hypertrophy of the inferior turbinate: long-term results in 382 patients randomly assigned to therapy. Ann Otol Rhinol Laryngol 1999;108(6):569–75.

[20] Passali D, Passali FM, Damiani V, et al. Treatment of inferior turbinate hypertrophy: a randomized clinical trial. Ann Otol Rhinol Laryngol 2003;112(8):683–8.

[21] Lippert BM, Werner JA. Comparison of carbon dioxide and neodymium: yttrium-aluminum-garnet lasers in surgery of the inferior turbinate. Ann Otol Rhinol Laryngol 1997;106(12):1036–42.

[22] Lippert BM, Werner JA. Long-term results after laser turbinectomy. Lasers Surg Med 1998; 22(2):126–34.

[23] Temple RH, Timms MS. Blood loss reduction during laser turbinectomy. Rhinology 2001; 39(4):230–2.

[24] Vagnetti A, Gobbi E, Algieri GM, et al. Wedge turbinectomy: a new combined photocoagulative Nd:YAG laser technique. Laryngoscope 2000;110(6):1034–6.

[25] Sapci T, Sahin B, Karavus A, et al. Comparison of the effects of radiofrequency tissue ablation, CO2 laser ablation, and partial turbinectomy applications on nasal mucociliary functions. Laryngoscope 2003;113(3):514–9.

[26] Mittleman H. CO2 laser turbinectomies for chronic, obstructive rhinitis. Lasers Surg Med 1982;2(1):29–36.

[27] Elwany S, Abel Salaam S. Laser surgery for allergic rhinitis: the effect on seromucinous glands. Otolaryngol Head Neck Surg 1999;120(5):742–4.

[28] Elwany S, Harrison R. Inferior turbinectomy: comparison of four techniques. J Laryngol Otol 1990;104(3):206–9.

[29] Mladina R, Risavi R, Subaric M. CO2 laser anterior turbinectomy in the treatment of non-allergic vasomotor rhinopathia. A prospective study upon 78 patients. Rhinology 1991; 29(4):267–71.

[30] Kawamura S, Fukutake T, Kubo N, et al. Subjective results of laser surgery for allergic rhinitis. Acta Otolaryngol Suppl 1993;500:109–12.

[31] Fukutake T, Kumazawa T, Nakamura A. Laser surgery for allergic rhinitis. AORN J 1987; 46(4):756–61.

[32] Fukutake T, Yamashita T, Tomoda K, et al. Laser surgery for allergic rhinitis. Arch Otolaryngol Head Neck Surg 1986;112(12):1280–2.

[33] Levine HL. The potassium–titanyl phosphate laser for treatment of turbinate dysfunction. Otolaryngol Head Neck Surg 1991;104(2):247–51.

[34] Goldsher M, Joachims HZ, Golz A, et al. Nd:YAG laser turbinate surgery animal experimental study: preliminary report. Laryngoscope 1995;105(3 Pt 1):319–21.

[35] Lenz H, Eichler J, Schafer G, et al. Production of a nasoantral window with an Ar + -laser. J Maxillofac Surg 1977;5(4):314–7.

[36] Metson R. Holmium:YAG laser endoscopic sinus surgery: a randomized, controlled study. Laryngoscope 1996;106(1 Pt 2 Suppl 77):1–18.

[37] Woog JJ, Metson R, Puliafito CA. Holmium:YAG endonasal laser dacryocystorhinostomy. Am J Ophthalmol 1993;116(1):1–10.

[38] Metson R, Woog JJ, Puliafito CA. Endoscopic laser dacryocystorhinostomy. Laryngoscope 1994;104(3 Pt 1):269–74.

[39] Szubin L, Papageorge A, Sacks E. Endonasal laser-assisted dacryocystorhinostomy. Am J Rhinol 1999;13(5):371–4.

[40] Kong YT, Kim TI, Kong BW. A report of 131 cases of endoscopic laser lacrimal surgery. Ophthalmology 1994;101(11):1793–800.

[41] Ohyama M. Laser polypectomy. Rhinol Suppl 1989;8:35–43.

[42] Fong M, Clarke K, Cron C. Clinical applications of the holmium:YAG laser in disorders of the paediatric airway. J Otolaryngol 1999;28(6):337–43.

[43] Furuta S, Itoh K, Shima T, et al. Laser beam in treating congenital choanal atresia in three patients. Acta Otolaryngol Suppl 1994;517:33–5.

[44] Healy GB, McGill T, Jako GJ, et al. Management of choanal atresia with the carbon dioxide laser. Ann Otol Rhinol Laryngol 1978;87(5 Pt 1):658–62.

[45] Illum P. Congenital choanal atresia treated by laser surgery. Rhinology 1986;24(3):205–9.

[46] Meer A, Tschopp K. Choanal atresia in premature dizygotic twins–a transnasal approach with Holmium:YAG-laser. Rhinology 2000;38(4):191–4.

[47] Muntz HR. Pitfalls to laser correction of choanal atresia. Ann Otol Rhinol Laryngol 1987; 96(1 Pt 1):43–6.

[48] Panwar SS, Martin FW. Trans-nasal endoscopic holmium: YAG laser correction of choanal atresia. J Laryngol Otol 1996;110(5):429–31.

[49] Pototschnig C, Volklein C, Appenroth E, et al. Transnasal treatment of congenital choanal atresia with the KTP laser. Ann Otol Rhinol Laryngol 2001;110(4):335–9.

[50] Tzifa KT, Skinner DW. Endoscopic repair of unilateral choanal atresia with the KTP laser: a one stage procedure. J Laryngol Otol 2001;115(4):286–8.

[51] Rothaug PG, Tulleners EP. Neodymium:yttrium-aluminum-garnet laser-assisted excision of progressive ethmoid hematomas in horses: 20 cases (1986–1996). J Am Vet Med Assoc 1999; 214(7):1037–41.

[52] Lund VJ, Howard DJ. A treatment algorithm for the management of epistaxis in hereditary hemorrhagic telangiectasia. Am J Rhinol 1999;13(4):319–22.
[53] Vickery CL, Kuhn FA. Using the KTP/532 laser to control epistaxis in patients with hereditary hemorrhagic telangiectasia. South Med J 1996;89(1):78–80.
[54] Mehta AC, Livingston DR, Levine HL. Fiberoptic bronchoscope and Nd-YAG laser in treatment of severe epistaxis from nasal hereditary hemorrhagic telangectasia and hemangioma. Chest 1987;91(5):791–2.
[55] Yu D, Ma Y, Xing Z. [Endoscopic surgery for nasal inverted papilloma]. Zhonghua Er Bi Yan Hou Ke Za Zhi 2001;36(3):169–71.
[56] Nakamura H, Kawasaki M, Higuchi Y, et al. Transnasal endoscopic resection of juvenile nasopharyngeal angiofibroma with KTP laser. Eur Arch Otorhinolaryngol 1999;256(4):212–4.
[57] Kronenberg J, Kessler A, Leventon G. Removal of a frontal sinus osteoma using the CO2 laser. Ear Nose Throat J 1986;65(10):480–1.

ELSEVIER
SAUNDERS

Otolaryngol Clin N Am
39 (2006) 503–522

OTOLARYNGOLOGIC
CLINICS
OF NORTH AMERICA

Computer Aided Surgery: Concepts and Applications in Rhinology

P. Daniel Knott, MD, Pete S. Batra, MD,
Martin J. Citardi, MD, FACS*

*The Cleveland Clinic Head and Neck Institute,
9500 Euclid Avenue, Cleveland, OH 44195, USA*

Computer-aided surgery (CAS), a technology developed in the 1980s and 1990s, has become relevant in a large and growing number of disciplines, including general surgery, neurosurgery, orthopedic surgery, otorhinolaryngology–head and neck surgery, and plastic surgery. In 1996, the International Society for Computer-Aided Surgery (ISCAS) defined the scope of CAS, as encompassing "all fields within surgery, as well as biomedical imaging and instrumentation, and digital technology employed as adjunct to imaging in diagnosis, therapeutics, and surgery" [1]. The vast domain of CAS includes surgical navigation, virtual reality, computer-aided image review, stereotactic surgery, robotic surgery, telemedicine, computer-aided tumor modeling, and many other applications. Within the field of otorhinolaryngology–head and neck surgery, CAS has had a major impact on functional endoscopic sinus surgery (FESS) and minimally invasive endoscopic skull base surgery. Image-guided surgery (IGS) has emerged as the term that describes intraoperative surgical navigation in otorhinolaryngology; thus, IGS is a type of CAS.

Recognition of complications resulting from inappropriate use of the endoscopic techniques within the complicated three-dimensional anatomy of the nasal cavity and paranasal sinuses spurred the development of surgical navigation systems. CAS acts as enabling technology by facilitating the surgeon's understanding of the relevant anatomy. Technological developments

---

Dr. Citardi was a member of the scientific advisory board of CBYON (Mountain View, California) from 1999 to 2003. He currently is a member of the scientific advisory board of GE Healthcare Navigation & Visualization (Lawrence, Massachusetts).

Dr. Batra is a consultant for Critical Therapeutics, Inc. (Lexington, Massachusetts).

* Corresponding author.

E-mail address: citardm@ccf.org (M.J. Citardi).

within CAS, including preoperative image review, three-dimensional modeling, virtual reality, image-enhanced endoscopy, and other techniques, all serve to support comprehension of the surgical relationships between a lesion (or diseased tissue) and surrounding anatomic structures. Thus, CAS provides surgeons with greater precision and confidence through the stages of preoperative planning and intraoperative execution.

History

Although the precise origin of sinonasal navigation is uncertain, its modern history can be traced to Mosher, who measured the distances and angles within the nasal cavity and paranasal sinuses, and detailed the risks of inaccurate intranasal navigation [2]. Although relatively rudimentary, this anatomic study represented an initial attempt to define intraoperatively the limits of the nasal cavity and paranasal sinuses, and most importantly to provide the surgeon with a rough guide for safe surgical intervention. Although the teaching of these techniques was exceedingly difficult, intranasal sinus surgery was performed rarely until the 1970s and 1980s, when interest was rekindled [3]. The introduction of endoscopic surgery led to a dramatic increase in minimally invasive sinus surgery, but as these novel surgical techniques were being offered and practiced by a new generation of otorhinolaryngologists, complication rates increased [3–7].

Kennedy surveyed the American Academy of Otolaryngology regarding the elevated rate of complications following endoscopic sinus surgery and reported a 0.49% overall complication rate, which was likely a conservative estimate given the subjective nature of the survey [8]. Several studies found major endoscopic surgical complication rates ranging from 0% to 8% and the presence of a steep learning curve associated with endoscopic techniques [4–6].

CAS therefore was developed to provide surgeons with greater confidence with intraoperative decision making and to facilitate minimally invasive procedures. Initial forays into surgical navigation took place within the neurosurgical specialty. In 1976, Bergstrom and Greitz devised a plastic helmet-like appliance with a metal ring, which could be worn in a CT scanner and intraoperatively, providing a frame of reference for the surgical procedure [9]. This was followed in subsequent years by various head frames that provided a rigid box from which intraoperative navigation information could be derived. Experiments in frameless stereotaxy by Roberts, Watanabe, and others took place in the 1980s and 1990s [10,11]. The Aachen group (University of Technology and University Hospital, Aachen, Germany) performed many of the initial experiments in CAS within the field of otolaryngology–head and neck surgery. This group developed a stereotactic navigation arm based upon the use of potentiometers. Outcomes with this device and other devices and subsequent modifications were reported repeatedly in the literature; key findings included reduced operative risks, a clinical accuracy of 1 to 2 mm, and simplification of complex maneuvers (such as bone cuts for osteoplastic procedures) [12–15].

In the early and mid 1990s, Fried reported an initial clinical series that described the application of the InstaTrak system (Visualization Technology, now part of GE Visualization & Navigation, Lawrence, Massachusetts), a navigation platform that featured electromagnetic tracking and automatic image-to-patient registration [16]. Over the subsequent years, numerous publications described other systems and numerous applications within rhinology [3,17–22].

Hardware issues

Although CAS vendors tend to highlight the unique features of their specific systems, all IGS system share certain common features. The hardware for intraoperative navigation includes a computer workstation, a tracking system, and specific surgical instruments.

The computer workstation is the central component, because it supports the software that drives the entire process. The computer features a method for importing preoperative imaging data (typically through a computer network or digital media). The computer workstation runs software capable of rapidly performing the complicated algorithms of intra-operative navigation. In particular, the software must use the preoperative imaging data set (axial images) and render additional images (coronal and sagittal images, plus others). The software must incorporate positional information provided by the tracking system and display this information relative to the preoperative imaging data set.

The tracking system also has been termed a digitizer, because it digitizes three-dimensional space. In essence, this device allows precise tracking of instrument positions. A component that is attached to an instrument for positional information is called an intraoperative localization device (ILD). To compensate for changes in patient positioning, an ILD also is attached to the patient; this ILD is known as a dynamic reference frame (DRF), an indirect reference to fixed stereotaxy systems that require a rigid frame bolted to the patient. Of course, the DRF must be attached securely to the patient, and the relationship between the DRF and the surgical field must not be altered.

Currently available navigation systems use optical or electromagnetic digitizers. Early systems used electromechanical arms, but these have fallen from favor. In addition, acoustical systems are theoretically feasible; however, the noisy environment of the operating room makes them impractical.

Optical tracking

Optical tracking systems employ infrared emitters and receivers that track in real time the varying position of surgical instruments within the operative field. Active systems are configured with cameras that track the position of light emitting diodes (LEDs) on the DRF and on the ILDs. Passive systems include infrared light emitters that detect the infrared light reflected from highly reflective spheres of the ILD (Fig. 1) mounted on the DRF and the calibrated instruments. In either case, the tracking system triangulates the position of the ILDs and sends this information to the navigation software. Unique arrangements of LEDs (or reflective spheres) on the ILD array gives each ILD a unique optical signature; thus, optical tracking systems can track three to six ILDs at any time.

The primary advantages of optical tracking systems are that virtually any calibrated instrument may be used for navigation, and that submillimetric accuracy may be achieved, at least in the laboratory setting. Although attaching a passive optical ILD to an instrument was somewhat cumbersome in the past, newer systems employ simplified designs to facilitate this step (Fig. 2). Disadvantages include the need for an uninterrupted visual axis between the ILDs and the overhead camera arrays.

Electromagnetic

Electromagnetic (EM) tracking systems employ an electromagnetic transmitter mounted on a headset worn by the patient at the time of the surgical procedure (Fig. 3). Receivers then are incorporated into specialized instruments, such as suction tips, which may be used to verify intraoperative accuracy and guide the dissection.

EM tracking eliminates the need for maintenance of an optical axis. Only specially designed instruments, however, may be calibrated and used for navigation. The potential also exists for disruption of the electromagnetic signal by an excess of metal in the immediate vicinity of the patient, although software design and hardware modifications may mitigate this effect.

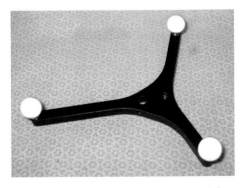

Fig. 1. This representative intraoperative localization device (ILD) features three highly reflective spheres that reflect light from an overhead infrared emitter to a camera array that can calculate instrument position. Active ILDs use light-emitting diodes (LEDs) in place of the reflective spheres.

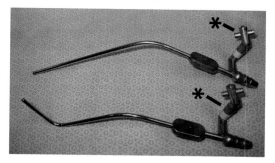

Fig. 2. Surgical instruments must incorporate a tracking device for intraoperative localization. These suctions featurè an offset post, indicated by "*", which is used to attach an intraoperative localization device.

Registration principles

Once imaging data have been uploaded into the IGS platforms, these data must be correlated with the physical data in the operating room. Using a process known as registration, the IGS platform calculates a mapping relationship between coordinates in the imaging space and the physical space, such that points in the two spaces that correspond to the same anatomical point are mapped to each other. Protocols for registration may be classified

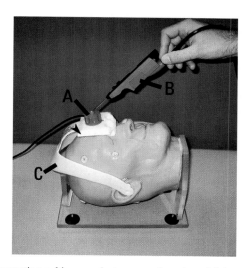

Fig. 3. For electromagnetic tracking, an electromagnetic emitter (A) is attached to the patient, and the surgical tool (B) incorporates a receiver that senses position relative to the electromagnetic field generated by the emitter. The headset (C) is used to secure the emitter to the patient. This headset (InstaTrak, GE Healthcare Navigation & Visualization, Lawrence, Massachusetts) also contains fiducial markers that permit automatic registration. The arrow head points to one of these markers.

into three broad categories called paired point registration (PPR), automatic registration, and contour-based registration (CBR). A common misconception is that the tracking system determines the registration protocol. In reality, engineers may choose to pair any registration protocol with any tracking system during the development of a system. Of course, commercially available systems are designed to support specific registration protocols, but in their development phase, almost any combination had been possible.

Registration must not be confused with calibration, which is the process of defining the position of an instrument tip relative to a tracking device.

Paired point registration

PPR represents the earliest and most basic form of registration. PPR involves the individual determination of the three-dimensional coordinates of corresponding fiducial points in the image and physical spaces, and then the calculation (by the computer software) of the transformation that best aligns these points. Anatomical landmarks may be used, or fiducial markers may be bone-anchored or skin-affixed. Anatomical landmark PPR, known as landmark registration, takes advantage of the discrete three-dimensional anatomical features of the human face, such as the tragus, medial canthus, lateral canthus, and nasal tip, by essentially using these features as fiducial markers. Although this registration method is simple, small but unavoidable differences in relative landmark positions caused by soft tissue deformation, changes in levels of tissue hydration, and inaccurate landmark localization may result in unacceptably large registration errors. Bone-anchored fiducial markers have been demonstrated to offer the greatest intraoperative accuracy (mean 1.0 mm $\pm$ 0.5 SD), although they are not necessarily significantly better than skin-affixed markers [23,24]. Although of experimental interest, the use of bone-anchored markers is simply not feasible, except in cases where ultraprecise targeting is critical. Skin-affixed fiducial markers are easy to place, but their use may be limited, as displacement before the subsequent operative procedure necessitates repeated image acquisition, and skin-affixed markers demonstrate a surprisingly amount of mobility.

The paired points used in this paradigm represent the same fiducial marker that must be localized on the preoperative imaging data set and on the patient at the start of the procedure. The surgeon must locate each point in the imaging data set manually and then pair it with the corresponding marker in the physical space, using a properly calibrated probe. Greatest precision is achieved when orthogonal images are available. After a series of these fiducial points are localized, the IGS platform software calculates the registration, which is basically a transformational algorithm.

Automatic registration

Automatic registration represents a variation of PPR. Fiducial markers are incorporated into the semirigid plastic head frames used in certain systems (InstaTrak; CBYON, Med-Surgical, Mountain View, California) (Fig. 3). For automatic registration, the patient must wear this headset at the time of preoperative imaging and at the time of surgery. The relative positions of the fiducial markers are defined, and the software can recognize the markers in the preoperative imaging study automatically and thus establish a relationship between the fiducial markers and the patient in the preoperative imaging. Because the head frame is designed to fit each patient in only one way, a patient may wear the head frame during image acquisition and subsequently during the operative procedure, without significant drift in the position of the fiducial markers. At the time of surgery, the computer workstation automatically localizes the fiducial markers on the headset and calculates a registration match.

Advantages of automatic registration include ease of use, rapid registration, and freedom from concern about fiducial displacement or dislodgement. Disadvantages of automatic registration include the potential for headset repositioning error, if the headset is not worn in exactly the same way during image acquisition and the operative procedure, and an inability to alter to fiducial configuration to suit a particular surgical procedure. When used appropriately, automatic registration greatly simplifies registration.

Contour-based registration

CBR, the newest registration protocol, has gathered increasing interest over the past several years. Imaging data are loaded onto the IGS platform, which constructs a virtual three-dimensional model based upon the surface contours of the images. In the operating room, the physical contours of the patients' facial anatomy must be loaded into the IGS platform, using either a calibrated hand-held probe, which is used to trace soft-tissue contours of underlying bony anatomy, or a hand-held laser, which is used to reflect light off of the contours of a patient's face to overhead cameras. A multitude of discrete points (125 to 500) are localized. The workstation completes the registration by calculating the best alignment of the preoperative imaging data set and the intraoperative contour-based point cloud by means of an iterative software algorithm. Laser registration has been found to be significantly faster than surface touch registration (20 versus 63 seconds, $P < .05$), although accuracy was equivalent for the two systems in the range of 2 mm) [25]. Another study on laser registration showed mean accuracy of 2.4 ± 1.7 mm, although the range of accuracy was large (1 to 9 mm) [26].

So-called mask registration, now part of the Stryker Navigation System (Stryker-Leibinger, Kalamazoo, Michigan) is really a variation of CBR. In this approach, the patient wears a flexible mask that contains multiple LEDs at the time of surgery. The overhead camera array localizes the position of these LEDs, and this positional information then defines contours that support CBR.

The primary advantage of CBR is the avoidance of headsets at the time of image acquisition. It also eliminates errors associated with fiducial localization. On the other hand, this approach may be inaccurate if surface contours are altered between the time of image acquisition and actual registration. Furthermore, CBR relies upon statistical assumptions that the recorded points accurately characterize a contour; although this may be true over a large number of patients, CBR is prone to instances of poor registration accuracy in individual cases.

Registration error

Registration error theory, which was developed for PPR, defines three types of error: fiducial localization error (FLE), fiducial registration error (FRE), and target registration error (TRE) [23]. Although the concepts for FLE, FRE, and TRE apply strictly only to PPR, they have important implications for automatic registration and CBR.

Fiducial localization error

FLE is the difference between the true position of a fiducial marker in the physical space and its measured position on preoperative images on the IGS platform. Point-based registration usually is performed with multiple fiducial markers (usually more than six to seven) and each individual fiducial marker will have an independent FLE. FLE usually is presented as the root mean square (RMS) average of the localization error, which is the square root of its expected squared value (ie, RMS [FLE] = $\sqrt{(FLE^2)}$). FLE depends on several factors, including the type of position sensor and the number, configuration, and type of fiducial markers employed [27]. Within the image space, factors that influence FLE include the shape and size of the fiducial marker, the voxel dimensions of the image, the digital intensity of the image, the contrast of the fiducial relative to its background in the image, and the geometrical distortion of the image [23,27] All of these factors contribute to overall mean FLE error, which is not displayed by IGS platforms. FLE cannot be measured directly, but must be derived from fiducial registration error based upon Sibson's relationship [28].

Fiducial registration error

FRE is the distance, after registration, between the measured position of a fiducial in the physical space and its measured position in the image space (ie, the residual error between fiducial points that are used for navigation after alignment). FRE can refer to the registration error of an individual fiducial, but FRE usually represents the mean RMS average of the individual registration errors. FRE is the only quantity directly measurable by IGS platforms. Clinical experience dictates that lower RMS is associated with better overall accuracy, although this is not necessarily true in every individual case.

Target registration error

TRE is the distance, after registration, between the position of a surgical target in the image space and its true position within the surgical field. This last measurement is the most relevant, as it represents a real-world accuracy measurement encountered every time a surgeon confirms the position of a target against the IGS platform imaging. TRE indicates how accurately the system tracks the positions of various calibrated instruments within the volume of surgical interest. Thus, TRE is the error of direct surgical interest. In the clinical realm, it can be determined by the surgeon only by reviewing localizations against known anatomic structures.

Although FLE, FRE, and TRE are vector quantities, they usually are represented as scalar values that represent the lengths of the vectors, without giving the direction of the error. During surgery, the surgeon may compensate for suboptimal navigation accuracy by noting the apparent vector of estimated TRE and compensating for it during subsequent localization against unknown targets.

Optimizing navigation accuracy

Finite errors made in the performance of registration will occur during any of the steps described, and will be compounded by errors made in subsequent steps during system set-up. Therefore, great attention must be directed to each step in the registration process, to optimize overall target accuracy. Certain strategies may be employed to minimize error.

Fiducial point selection

Each fiducial marker will have an inherent FLE during registration. Exclusion of individual fiducial points with high FLE has been shown to optimize subsequent accuracy [29]. Although IGS platforms may attempt to perform exclusion automatically, a high number of poorly localized fiducial points will result in unacceptable accuracy. Therefore, the imaging data set should be obtained with as thin a slice thickness as possible, and repeated attempts at localization may be required until an optimal TRE value is obtained. When performing PPR, great care must be exercised to obtain the best possible matching, as operator error may be a significant component of FLE. Therefore, the best results may be obtained when the most experienced team member performs the PPR.

Fiducial point number

Fiducial number is an important component of overall accuracy. Although the fiducial number is fixed with headset-based registration protocols, this number may be altered when using CBR, landmark-based PPR, or external fiducial marker PPR. Although the optimal number of fiducial points is not certain, general practice has been to use as many fiducial points as feasible. At least three fiducial points are required to generate a three-dimensional image transformation. Additional well-localized fiducial points will improve the registration accuracy, while poorly localized fiducial points may worsen registration accuracy. The optimal number of fiducial points in CBR recently was examined [30]. Using the InstaTrak 3500 Plus system, TRE was measured at two positions on the skull base using 500, 250, 125, 50, and 4 fiducial points for registration. TRE was optimized when 50 or 125 points were used, with mean accuracy and standard error worsening with the use of greater or fewer points.

Fiducial configuration

The borders of the high accuracy centroid (minimum mean x, y, z co-ordinate distance to all fiducial points; that is the center of the fiducial arrangement) are directly dependent on the shape of the fiducial configuration (Fig. 4). When collinear fiducial points are employed, the high accuracy zone is relatively shallow and small, with TRE increasing as target distance from the centroid increases [31,32]. This is obviously problematic when fiducial points are located anteriorly, and the surgical targets of interest are located posteriorly within the sinonasal cavity. With a noncollinear distribution of fiducial points, such as with a headset with a three-dimensional fiducial configuration or with CBR with points located in multiple different

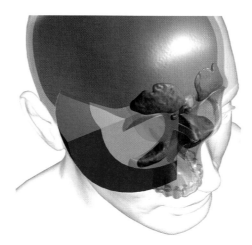

Fig. 4. The zones of anticipated greatest surgical navigational accuracy (low target registration error, TRE) are represented by a three-dimensional target. These zones reflect the characteristics of the registration for a specific case, and they may be calculated based upon principles derived from registration error theory. TRE will be greatest at the centroid, and thus, it is desirable for the centroid to be deep in the nasal cavity in the area that is closest to the greatest surgical challenges.

planes, the shape of the high-accuracy centroid may be enlarged and may be located more posteriorly. Therefore, to optimize TRE, fiducial points should be distributed symmetrically around the volume of surgical interest, such that the centroid is located as close to the area of surgical interest as possible [33].

Image acquisition

Preoperative images are acquired on either a CT or MRI scanner. The scanner performs a series of discrete slices or cuts of a subject in the axial plane with a determined thickness, from which coronal and sagittal reformats are created. These data then are stored in the form of two-dimensional pixels, which must be converted into voxels or three-dimensional arrays of elements. A voxel represents the average radiograph attenuation over the region covered by pixel in the planar images. Overall accuracy therefore is limited by the voxel resolution, for as voxel size increases, volume averaging will lead to a greater loss of anatomic detail. Currently, voxel sizes on the order of 1 mm are achieved routinely [23].

Navigational accuracy (target registration error)

Review of the CAS literature is confusing because of the lack of standardized nomenclature and methodology for determinations of navigational accuracy [34]. Furthermore, accuracy measurements will differ depending upon the location of the surgical target within the surgical field and upon the relationship between the target and the fiducial points. Therefore, comparisons of accuracy reports for the different systems are difficult. Table 1 provides a summary of accuracy for currently available CAS systems.

The most important aspect of CAS is the provision of accurate intraoperative navigation. Although the language used in the literature is variable, the term that is most synonymous with the surgeon's perception of intraoperative accuracy is TRE. Early systems tested with plastic or acrylic models yielded error measurements of approximately 2 mm [11,35,36]. True intraoperative TRE often is obtained in the range of 1 to 2 mm, which likely represents the reproducible practical limit of navigation accuracy with the current technology. Claims regarding superior accuracy may be made, but surgeons should regard these claims with caution, as the range of error may be quite high, leading to very poor accuracy with a subset of patients. In selected instances, intraoperative surgical navigation accuracy may be truly submillimetric; however, in other cases with the same system, the accuracy may be considerably worse (3 to 4 mm or worse). Thus, mean accuracy estimates and the range of accuracy measurements are both important. Intraoperative decision making should take into account the worst likely value of TRE, and therefore repeated referencing of accuracy against known anatomical landmarks is recommended [37].

Table 1
Reported target registration error for commercially available image-guided surgery platforms

System (vendor)	Tracking system	Registration type	Reported accuracy
InstaTrak (GE Navigation & Visualization Lawrence, MA)	Electromagnetic	Automatic	2.28mm (95% CI 2.02–2.53) [43]
		PPR	1.97mm (95% CI 1.75–2.23) [43]
		CBR with touch	1.5 +/− 0.3 mm [30]
Landmarx (Medtronic Xomed Jacksonville, FL)	Optical	Automatic	N/A
		PPR	1.69 +/− 0.38mm [21]
		CBR	No report
Stryker Navigation System (Stryker-Leibinger Kalamazoo, MI)	Optical	Automatic	N/A
		PPR	1.6mm (range 0.6–3.7) [29]
		CBR (mask)	No report
VectorVision (BrainLAB Hemstetten, Germany)	Optical	Automatic	No report
		PPR	1.57 +/− 1.1mm [47]
		CBR with laser	2.4 +/− 1.7mm [26]

Abbreviations: CBR, contour-based registration; N/A, registration protocol not available for the specific system; PPR, paired-point registration.

Current applications

The American Academy of Otolaryngology–Head and Neck Surgery has published an official policy statement on the indications for surgical navigation [38]. According to this statement, the use of this technology is at the discretion of the rhinologic surgeon. Specific indications include:

- Revision sinus surgery
- Traumatic, developmental, or postoperative anomalies
- Sinonasal polyposis
- Surgery for frontal, posterior ethmoidal, and sphenoidal sinus disease
- Lesions adjacent to the skull base, orbit, optic nerve, or carotid artery
- Cerebrospinal fluid rhinorrhea
- Benign and malignant sinonasal neoplasms

CAS should be incorporated into FESS technique to create a paradigm for IG-FESS [19]. In this strategy, CAS is an enabling technology that facilitates the comprehension of complex three-dimensional relationships and compensates for the perceptual distortion intrinsic to visualization provided by surgical telescopes. For maximal benefit, the surgeon should use the CAS system interactively preoperatively and intraoperatively, and the CAS should be configured with an appropriate user interface and instrumentation to support its easy use during surgery. IG-FESS is suited best for the most complicated surgical challenges, including frontal sinus surgery (Fig. 5), posterior ethmoid and sphenoid surgery (Fig. 6), revision surgery (Figs. 7, 8), and sinonasal polyposis, allergic fungal rhinosinusitis, and other applications.

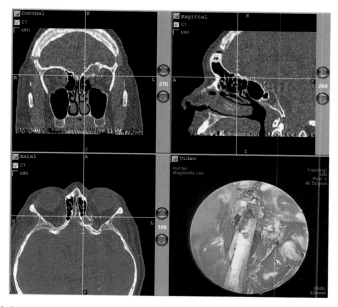

Fig. 5. This intraoperative screen capture shows the tip of the curved aspirator (as seen in the endoscopic image in the lower right panel) at the entrance to a post-traumatic mucocele in a supraorbital ethmoid cell. The opening of the supraorbital ethmoid cell was quite narrow, and surgical navigation greatly facilitated identification of the relevant landmarks.

Two recent developments have begun to extend the applications of CAS even further for minimally invasive approaches to the skull base. These developments provide better information about soft tissue anatomic relationships and the internal carotid artery (ICA):

CT–MRI fusion

IGS commonly is performed with CT imaging data, given the bony box represented by the nasal cavity and paranasal sinuses. Occasionally, MRI data are preferred when greater soft tissue detail is important, as in assessing dural involvement of a skull base tumor, or defining the limits of a pituitary tumor. CT–MRI fusion software performs an image-to-image registration between corresponding CT and MRI scans and then permits the display of fused image data that contain CT and MRI information. The CT–MRI fusion scan can be used for surgical navigation (Fig. 9). CT–MRI fusion technology enables a surgeon to pair the fine bony detail of CT imaging with the discrete soft-tissue information conveyed by MRI technology. Instead of using each data set independently, CT/MR merging protocols permit bone/soft tissue composite overlays to be created. The surgeon may toggle between the data sets or adjust the intensity of the relative images at any point along the spectrum between these two modalities. Similarly,

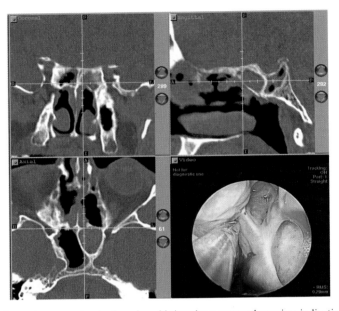

Fig. 6. Endoscopic approaches to the sphenoid sinus have emerged as prime indications for surgical navigation. In this intraoperative screen capture, the tip of the aspirator (in the endoscopic image in the lower right panel) is at the left sphenoid face.

CT or MRI data may be merged with positron emission tomography (PET) imaging data to provide anatomical and functional data, which may be particularly valuable when approaching sinus or skull base neoplasms by a minimally invasive technique. A recent report describes current applications for CT–MRI fusion in detail [39].

Three-dimensional CT angiography

Endoscopic approaches to the sphenoid sinus often are limited by an inability to precisely localize the position of the ICA at the skull base. Three-dimensional CT angiography (CTA) is software-driven process for rendering virtual angiography images of the contrast-filled ICA from rapid CT acquisition coordinated with a bolus of intravenous contrast (Fig. 10). Surgical navigation with three-dimensional CTA images facilitates the definition of the anatomic relationships between the skull base and the ICA [40].

Outcome studies

The introduction of expensive new technology such as CAS requires an analysis of its potential impact using principles of evidence-based medicine. Unfortunately, such an analysis is problematic for this surgical technology

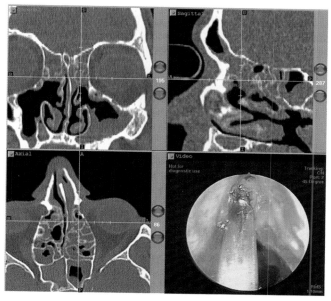

Fig. 7. Revision sinus surgery is another prime indication for surgical navigation. In this example, the aspirator (in the endoscopic image in the lower right panel) has been placed on residual ethmoid cells, which may be studied on the orthogonal CT views before intraoperative dissection.

(as it is for many other surgical technologies), because it is essentially impossible to design and implement a comprehensive study to address these issues. Nonetheless, the surgical literature and other anecdotal reports demonstrate the usefulness of CAS. In particular, multiple retrospective studies, which have employed as control groups patients having undergone sinus surgery without IGS, have demonstrated improvements in complication rates [3,21,41,42], but these differences have not been statistically significant. In one study that did show a statistically significant benefit, Fried found that the use of IGS technology enabled surgeons to treat more severe polyposis with fewer complications, and decreased the need for revision procedures within 3 months of the initial procedure [43].

The use of CAS systems has been shown to increase the mean operative time of cases. Although this effect is relatively large during the early learning curve, familiarity with the instrumentation has reduced this to approximately 15 minutes [3,21,44]. It is possible that reductions in operative time because of CAS may compensate for the extra time associated with CAS set-up and registration.

Economic implications

CAS technology is expensive, with most platform list prices starting at $150,000 or more, although models that feature less robust technology

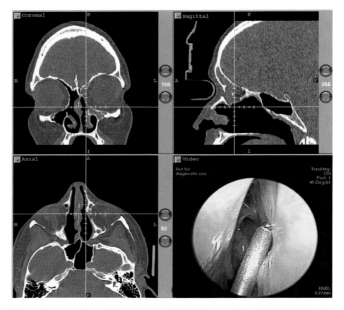

Fig. 8. In this patient, previous sinus surgery included resection of the left lamina papyracea, with secondary displacement of the orbital contents medially. Postoperatively, she developed left frontal headache because of a mucocele. During the revision procedure, surgical navigation was used to avoid the dehiscent orbital wall as the frontal mucocele was opened. In this screen capture, the aspirator tip (in the endoscopic image in the lower right panel) is on the dehiscent medial orbital wall.

may cost considerably less. Moreover, the technology is upgraded continuously, and, thus periodic, significant added costs are incurred to maintain the platform hardware and software. Also, even simple repairs will limit the use of the platform and increase the overall application costs. Metson and colleagues reported that the use of an IGS system increased hospital costs by $496 per case [21].

The 2000 revision of Current Procedural Terminology (CPT) amended the definition of CPT code 61795 to include extracranial applications, including rhinologic applications; however, reimbursement for this code is quite variable. Because of concerns about assuring availability of this technology, professional societies, such as the American Rhinologic Society, have taken a leadership role in reimbursement-related issues for CAS.

Future directions

Current IGS technology only enables a surgeon to navigate with images obtained before the surgical intervention. Although soft tissue deformation is limited in sinus surgery, the appeal of real-time imaging of the changing

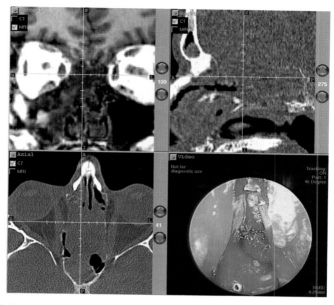

Fig. 9. This intraoperative screen capture shows localization along the anterior cranial fossa dura in a patient with a large esthesioneuroblastoma that was treated by preoperative chemotherapy and radiation therapy followed by computer-aided minimally invasive endoscopic resection. For this case, an image-to-image registration was performed to fuse the preoperative CT and MRI scans, and then a standard image-to-patient registration was completed for surgical navigation. In this image capture, the upper left panel is an MRI scan, the bottom right image is the endoscopic image, and the remaining quadrants are conventional CT images.

intraoperative anatomy during the course of the procedure is clear. Attempts at developing intraoperative imaging have been limited by the cost and cumbersome nature of the technology, although Fried found that the use of real-time MRI may have some utility, particularly when soft-tissue detail is essential [45]. The development of smaller, more powerful magnets and greater automation within the operating room may make this technology more feasible in the future. The use of real time CT scanning has not been a great option, in light of concerns about radiation exposure and poor image quality, but future developments may obviate these concerns. In theory, near real-time updates could be achieved through the use of intraoperative CT scanners. The use of fluoroscopy-derived tomographic images (with near CT image quality) for surgical navigation has been reported [46].

Recent technological advances, such as CBR, three-dimensional CTA and CT–MRI fusion, have been grafted onto previously introduced CAS platforms. As a result, the integration of these new developments into the surgical workflow has been problematic. Thus, it is hoped that the next generation of platforms will feature an improved interface that supports

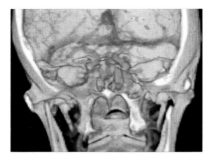

Fig. 10. This screen capture illustrates the path of each internal carotid artery (ICA) at the skull base as depicted in this image rendered through three-dimensional CT angiography. By scrolling through the images sequentially, it is possible to trace the path of the ICA relative to the skull base and skull base pathology.

simple implementation of routine navigation, but also better integrates the advanced applications.

Summary

Although CAS was conceived initially as adjunctive technology, developments, refinements, and its acceptance have made it into a transformative technology with many applications within rhinology and other surgical disciplines. For reliable routine use of IGS, surgeons should develop a working familiarity with registration error theory so that they can minimize the significant risks resulting from inaccurate navigation. Today, CAS is used routinely for the most complex cases treated by FESS and for minimally invasive, endoscopic approaches to the skull base. Both three-dimensional CTA and CT–MRI fusion have been incorporated recently into CAS and may further extend the surgical application. Reported clinical experiences suggest that although CAS is not required for every case, it does offer significant advantages for the most complex cases (eg, revision surgery, frontal sinus, sphenoid and posterior ethmoid, sinonasal polyposis, and tumors). Nonetheless, CAS is not a substitute for vigorous surgical training, knowledge of surgical anatomy, and sound intraoperative surgical decision making. Improvements in technology may lead to further improvements in accuracy, reliability, and utility. Thus, CAS has emerged as important component for advanced rhinologic surgical techniques.

References

[1] International Society for Computer-Aided Surgery. Computer-aided surgery: aims and scope. Available at: www.iscas.net/. Accessed November 26, 2005.
[2] Mosher HP. Measurements for operating distances in the nose. Ann Surg 1902;36:554–9.

[3] Reardon EJ. Navigational risks associated with sinus surgery and the clinical effects of implementing a navigational system for sinus surgery. Laryngoscope 2002;112:1–19.

[4] Stankiewicz JA. Complications of endoscopic intranasal ethmoidectomy. Laryngoscope 1987;97:1270–3.

[5] Stankiewicz JA. Complications in endoscopic intranasal ethmoidectomy: an update. Laryngoscope 1989;99:686–90.

[6] Maniglia AJ. Fatal and other major complications of endoscopic sinus surgery. Laryngoscope 1991;101:349–54.

[7] May M, Levine HL, Mester SJ, et al. Complications of endoscopic sinus surgery: analysis of 2108 patients–incidence and prevention. Laryngoscope 1994;104:1080–3.

[8] Kennedy DW, Shaman P, Han W, et al. Complications of ethmoidectomy: a survey of fellows of the American Academy of Otolaryngology-Head and Neck Surgery. Otolaryngol Head Neck Surg 1994;111:589–99.

[9] Bergstrom M, Greitz T. Stereotaxic computed tomography. AJR Am J Roentgenol 1976; 127:167–70.

[10] Roberts DW, Strohbehn JW, Hatch JF, et al. A frameless stereotaxic integration of computerized tomographic imaging and the operating microscope. J Neurosurg 1986;65: 545–9.

[11] Watanabe E, Watanabe T, Manaka S, et al. Three-dimensional digitizer (neuronavigator): new equipment for computed tomography-guided stereotaxic surgery. Surg Neurol 1987; 27:543–7.

[12] Carrau RL, Snyderman CH, Curtin HB, et al. Computer-assisted frontal sinusotomy. Otolaryngol Head Neck Surg 1994;111:727–32.

[13] Anon JB, Lipman SP, Oppenheim D, et al. Computer-assisted endoscopic sinus surgery. Laryngoscope 1994;104:901–5.

[14] Klimek L, Mosges R, Schlondorff G, et al. Development of computer-aided surgery for otorhinolaryngology. Comput Aided Surg 1998;3:194–201.

[15] Klimek L, Ecke U, Lubben B, et al. A passive-marker-based optical system for computer-aided surgery in otorhinolaryngology: development and first clinical experiences. Laryngoscope 1999;9:1509–15.

[16] Fried MP, Kleefield J, Gopal H, et al. Image-guided endoscopic surgery: results of accuracy and performance in a multicenter clinical study using an electromagnetic tracking system. Laryngoscope 1997;107:594–601.

[17] Anon JB, Klimek L, Mosges R, et al. Computer-assisted endoscopic sinus surgery. An international review. Otolaryngol Clin North Am 1997;30:389–401.

[18] Anon JB. Computer-aided endoscopic sinus surgery. Laryngoscope 1998;108:949–61.

[19] Olson G, Citardi MJ. Image-guided functional endoscopic sinus surgery. Otolaryngol Head Neck Surg 2000;123:188–94.

[20] Metson R, Gliklich RE, Cosenza M. A comparison of image guidance systems for sinus surgery. Laryngoscope 1998;108:1164–70.

[21] Metson R, Cosenza M, Gliklich RE, et al. The role of image-guidance systems for head and neck surgery. Arch Otolaryngol Head Neck Surg 1999;125:1100–4.

[22] Metson RB, Cosenza MJ, Cunningham MJ, et al. Physician experience with an optical image guidance system for sinus surgery. Laryngoscope 2000;110:972–6.

[23] Maurer CR Jr, Rohlfing T, Dean D, et al. Sources of error in image registration for cranial image-guided neurosurgery. In: Germano IM, editor. Advanced techniques in image-guided brain and spine surgery. New York: Thieme; 2002. p. 10–36.

[24] Ammirati M, Gross JD, Ammirati G, et al. Comparison of registration accuracy of skin and bone implanted fiducials for frameless stereotaxis of the brain, a prospective study. Skull Base 2002;12:125–31.

[25] Woodworth BA, Davis GW, Schlosser RJ. Comparison of laser vs. surface touch registration for image-guided sinus surgery. Presented at the American Rhinologic Society 2005 Spring Meeting. Boca Raton (FL), May 13–14, 2005.

[26] Raabe A, Krishnan R, Wolff R, et al. Laser surface scanning for patient registration in intracranial image-guided surgery. Neurosurgery 2002;50:797–801 [discussion 802–3].

[27] West JB, Fitzpatrick JM, Toms SA, et al. Fiducial point placement and the accuracy of point-based, rigid body registration. Neurosurgery 2001;48:810–6 [discussion 816–7].

[28] Sibson R. Studies in the robustness of multi-dimensional scaling: perturbational analysis of classical scaling. Journal Review of Statistical Society 1979;41:213–25.

[29] Snyderman C, Zimmer LA, Kassam A. Sources of registration error with image guidance systems during endoscopic anterior cranial base surgery. Otolaryngol Head Neck Surg 2004;131:145–9.

[30] Knott PD, Batra PS, Butler RS, et al. Contour-based & paired-point registration in a model for image-guided surgery. Presented at the American Academy of Otolaryngology–Head and Neck Surgery 2005 Annual Meeting. Los Angeles (CA), September 25–28, 2005.

[31] Helm PA, Eckel TS. Accuracy of registration methods in frameless stereotaxis. Comput Aided Surg 1998;3:51–6.

[32] Knott PD, Maurer CR, Gallivan R, et al. The impact of fiducial distribution on headset-based registration in image-guided sinus surgery. Otolaryngol Head Neck Surg 2004;131: 666–72.

[33] Berry J, O'Malley BW Jr, Humphries S, et al. Making image guidance work: understanding control of accuracy. Ann Otol Rhinol Laryngol 2003;112:689–92.

[34] Labadie RF, Davis BM, Fitzpatrick JM. Image-guided surgery: what is the accuracy? Curr Opin Otolaryngol Head Neck Surg 2005;13:27–31.

[35] Watanabe E, Mayanagi Y, Kosugi Y, et al. Open surgery assisted by the neuronavigator, a stereotactic, articulated, sensitive arm. Neurosurgery 1991;28:792–9 [discussion 799–800].

[36] Zinreich SJ, Tebo SA, Long DM, et al. Frameless stereotaxic integration of CT imaging data: accuracy and initial applications. Radiology 1993;3:735–42.

[37] Caversaccio M, Zulliger D, Bachler R, et al. Practical aspects for optimal registration (matching) on the lateral skull base with an optical frameless computer-aided pointer system. Am J Otol 2000;21:863–70.

[38] American Academy of Otolaryngology–Head & Neck Surgery. AAO-HNS Policy on Intraoperative Use of Computer-Aided Surgery. Available at: www.entlink.net/practice/rules/image-guiding.cfm. Accessed November 26, 2005.

[39] Leong JL, Batra PS, Citardi MJ. CT–MR fusion for the management of skull base lesions. Presented the American Academy of Otolaryngology–Head and Neck Surgery 2005 Annual Meeting. Los Angeles (CA), September 25–28, 2005.

[40] Leong JL, Batra PS, Citardi MJ. Imaging of the internal carotid artery and adjacent skull base with three-dimensional CT angiography for preoperative planning and intraoperative surgical navigation. Laryngoscope 2005;115:1618–23.

[41] Sindwani R, Metson R. Impact of image guidance on complications during osteoplastic frontal sinus surgery. Otolaryngol Head Neck Surg 2004;131:150–5.

[42] Kacker A, Tabaee A, Anand V. Computer-assisted surgical navigation in revision endoscopic sinus surgery. Otolaryngol Clin North Am 2005;38:473–82.

[43] Fried MP, Moharir VM, Shin J, et al. Comparison of endoscopic sinus surgery with and without image guidance. Am J Rhinol 2002;16:193–7.

[44] Metson R. Intraoperative image-guidance technology. Arch Otolaryngol Head Neck Surg 1999;125:1278–9.

[45] Fried MP, Topulos G, Hsu L, et al. Endoscopic sinus surgery with magnetic resonance imaging guidance: initial patient experience. Otolaryngol Head Neck Surg 1998;119:374–80.

[46] Brown SM, Sadoughi BCH, Fried MP. Feasibility of real-time image-guided sinus surgery using intraoperative fluoroscopy. Presented at the American Rhinologic Society 2005 Annual Meeting. Los Angeles (CA), September 24, 2005.

[47] Cartellieri M, Kremser J, Vorbeck F. Comparison of different 3D navigation systems by a clinical user. Eur Arch Otorhinolaryngol 2001;258:38–41.

ELSEVIER
SAUNDERS

Otolaryngol Clin N Am
39 (2006) 523–538

OTOLARYNGOLOGIC
CLINICS
OF NORTH AMERICA

Endoscopic Management of Cerebrospinal Fluid Rhinorrhea

Rodney J. Schlosser, MD[a],*,
William E. Bolger, MD, FACS[b]

[a]Department of Otolaryngology–Head and Neck Surgery,
Medical University of South Carolina, 135 Rutledge Avenue, Suite 1130, PO Box 250550,
Charleston, SC 29425, USA
[b]Department of Surgery (Otolaryngology), Uniformed Services University of the Health
Sciences, 4301 Jones Bridge Road, Bethesda, MD 20814, USA

History

Transcranial repair of cerebrospinal fluid (CSF) leak was first reported by Dandy, who closed a cranionasal fistula via frontal craniotomy in 1926. The first extracranial approach was described in 1948 by Dohlman, who used a naso-orbital incision to close an anterior skull base CSF leak. Transnasal approaches subsequently were used by Hirsch in 1952 and Vrabec and Hallberg in 1964. Improved instrumentation for sinus surgery led to the endoscopic repair of CSF leaks by Wigand in 1981. Since the 1980s, the minimally invasive endoscopic approach has gained widespread acceptance. The diagnostic aspects and surgical techniques have evolved, leading to higher success rates (approximately 90%) and lower morbidity than traditional intracranial techniques for most leaks. The endoscopic approach has become the standard of care [1,2].

Normal physiology

It is helpful to understand normal CSF physiology to diagnose and treat patients with CSF rhinorrhea properly. CSF is formed primarily in the choroid plexus within the lateral, third, and fourth ventricles at a rate of 0.35 mL/min (20 mL/h or 350–500 mL/d). The total volume of CSF in an adult is approximately 90 to 150 mL; the total volume of CSF is turned over three to five times each day [3].

---

* Corresponding author.
E-mail address: schlossr@musc.edu (R.J. Schlosser).

0030-6665/06/$ - see front matter © 2006 Elsevier Inc. All rights reserved.
doi:10.1016/j.otc.2006.01.001

After production in the choroid plexus, CSF flows from the ventricular system into the subarachnoid space around the spinal cord and cerebral convexities. CSF absorption occurs along these convexities at the arachnoid villi. The villi project into the dural sinuses and act as one-way valves that typically require a pressure gradient of 1.5 to 7 cm H_2O for antegrade flow from the subarachnoid space into the dural sinuses. At lower pressure differentials, the villi close and prevent retrograde flow.

Normal CSF pressure is approximately 5 to 15 cm H_2O recorded in the lumbar cistern with the patient lying in the decubitus position. This pressure varies significantly depending on time of day, patient age, activity level, and cardiac and respiratory cycles. Neurologic symptoms may develop when pressures exceed 15 to 20 cm H_2O, and treatment to reduce intracranial pressure (ICP) generally is recommended for patients with mild-to-moderate elevations, even in the absence of symptoms [3].

Pathophysiology

Overview

CSF leaks can be categorized based on a variety of factors, such as etiology, anatomic site, or underlying ICP. The authors typically classify leaks based on etiology because this is usually apparent from the patient's clinical history, then take into account the impact that anatomic location and underlying ICP have on the surgical repair. All of these factors should be considered because they influence medical and surgical treatment and long-term success.

Accidental trauma

Historically, closed head injury secondary to accidental trauma is the most common etiology of CSF leaks. Leaks occur in approximately 1% to 3% of all closed head injuries (Fig. 1). These leaks usually begin within 2 days of the injury [4]. More than 70% close with observation or conservative treatment, such as bed rest or lumbar drain, but these nonsurgical closures probably result in closure with thin fibrous tissue or mucosa because dura mater does not regenerate [5]. Nonsurgical treatment has been associated with a significant incidence of ascending meningitis (30–40%) in long-term follow-up, despite leak cessation. More aggressive, early endoscopic repair may have a role in reducing this long-term risk of meningitis. Accidental traumatic CSF leaks are heterogeneous, and bony skull base defects can vary from a narrow crack in a blunt head injury, to multiple, comminuted cracks in projectile injuries.

Surgical trauma

The most common surgeries leading to iatrogenic skull base defects are functional endoscopic sinus surgery and neurologic surgery. Differences

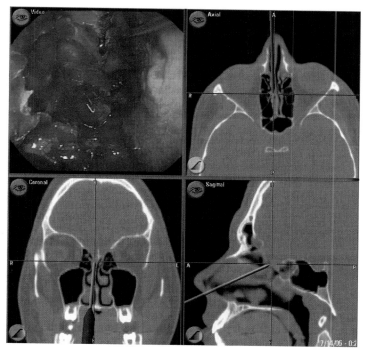

Fig. 1. Triplanar imaging of a closed head injury that resulted in a CSF leak and crack of the skull base that extended from the posterior table of the right frontal sinus to the face of the sphenoid along the olfactory cleft.

between accidental and surgical trauma may be the size of the bony defect and the degree of dural and associated brain parenchymal disruption. Iatrogenic defects typically occur during bone resection, often with powered instrumentation, and may result in bony defects 2 cm in size.

The two most common sites of skull base injury associated with functional endoscopic sinus surgery are the lateral lamella of the cribriform plate and the posterior ethmoid roof near the face of the sphenoid. Injury to the lateral lamella of the cribriform can occur during an approach to the anterior ethmoid or frontal recess or when resecting the middle turbinate close to the skull base (Fig. 2). The bone of the lateral lamella of the cribriform is usually thinner than the ethmoid roof and more susceptible to injury.

Iatrogenic posterior ethmoid defects typically occur in cases in which the maxillary sinus is highly pneumatized and expands superomedially, causing a corresponding and relative decrease in posterior ethmoid pneumatization. The superior-to-inferior dimension of the posterior ethmoid is reduced, narrowing the available surgical space before encountering the skull base.

CSF leak following neurologic surgery can occur after a variety of procedures, but the most common is pituitary surgery [6]. Disruption of the

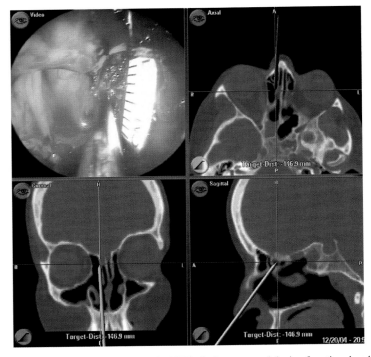

Fig. 2. Triplanar imaging of an iatrogenic CSF leak that occurred during functional endoscopic sinus surgery secondary to injury along the right lateral lamella.

sellar diaphragm by tumor or surgical trauma can result in a leak. Additionally, a misdirected approach for pituitary surgery that does not identify the sella properly can lead to an iatrogenic skull base defect. Other causes of CSF leak during neurosurgery include craniofacial resection and transcranial approaches.

Tumors

Skull base tumors can lead to CSF leaks directly or indirectly. Direct tumor invasion across the anterior skull base can cause large defects with significantly diseased or missing bone surrounding the defect (Fig. 3). These tumors can be primary central nervous system neoplasms that extend into the nasal cavity, or, conversely, they may be sinonasal primaries that extend intracranially. Treatments for the tumor itself, such as surgery, radiation, or chemotherapy, can create a devascularized wound bed and skull base defect that is difficult to repair. Noncurative treatments that leave persistent tumor also may compromise CSF leak repair.

Conversely, tumors can lead indirectly to CSF leaks by obstructing CSF flow, resulting in hydrocephalus. Success in these cases usually requires

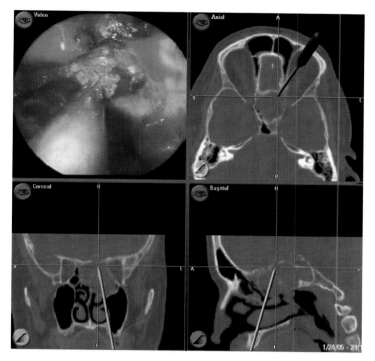

Fig. 3. Endoscopic resection of this large meningioma (triplanar imaging) resulted in a 2 × 3 cm skull base defect that was repaired endoscopically using soft tissue underlay and overlay grafts without the use of a lumbar drain.

treatment of the primary tumor to correct the obstruction or long-term shunting to divert the elevated CSF pressure. Repairing the CSF leak without treating the obstructing lesion may worsen the high-pressure condition because the internal relief valve for the patient's intracranial hypertension is removed.

Congenital

Congenital CSF leaks and encephaloceles are challenging to treat and are relatively rare. Our series showed that approximately 50% of congenital defects originate at the foramen cecum, and the other half occur in the vicinity of the cribriform plate or ethmoid roof [7]. These deformities typically are characterized by a funnel-shaped defect of the bony skull base through which a meningoencephalocele herniates into the sinonasal cavity. Surgical placement of epidural grafts can be difficult because of this misshapen, funnel-shaped skull base. Improved instrumentation has enabled repair of congenital encephaloceles at age 23 months [8]. ICPs in this group are generally normal, with the rare exception of patients with congenital hydrocephalus.

Similar to patients with hydrocephalus secondary to an obstructing tumor, the underlying high-pressure condition should be treated before definitive repair of the skull base defect.

Spontaneous

The authors' definition of spontaneous CSF leaks is limited to patients with no other discernible etiology for the CSF leak. Historically, a variety of clinical conditions have been classified as "spontaneous" CSF leaks, including leaks associated with tumor, delayed traumatic leaks, and leaks associated with congenital skull base malformation [9,10]. We believe CSF leaks that arise secondary to another condition (eg, tumor, trauma, congenital malformation) should be classified and described as such, even if the temporal history of leak occurrence is "spontaneous."

Clinical, radiographic, and demographic data suggest that spontaneous CSF leak patients represent a distinct clinical entity that is likely a variant of benign intracranial hypertension, and their elevated CSF pressures contribute to the development of CSF leaks [11]. Patients are most commonly middle-aged, obese women with pressure-type headaches, pulsatile tinnitus, and balance abnormalities in addition to their CSF rhinorrhea. Radiographically, they often have empty, expanded sellae, broadly attenuated skull bases, arachnoid pits, and multiple skull base defects secondary to chronic hydrostatic forces [12]. ICPs in these patients can be measured reliably via lumbar puncture or by using an indwelling lumbar drain and typically range from 15 to 52 cm H_2O [13]. Using the modified Dandy criteria and evaluating clinical, radiographic, and ICP data for the most rigid diagnosis of benign intracranial hypertension have shown that more than 70% of spontaneous leak patients meet the diagnostic criteria for benign intracranial hypertension (unpublished data). Of all etiologies for CSF leaks, the spontaneous group is associated with the highest rate (50–100%) of encephalocele formation, and there are often large meningoencephaloceles herniating through relatively small bony defects. Spontaneous leaks have the highest recurrence rate after surgical repair of the leak (25–87%) compared with less than 10% for most other etiologies [9,10,14]. Unfavorable conditions, such as elevated ICP, associated meningoencephaloceles, and broadly attenuated bony skull base undoubtedly contribute to this higher failure rate.

Preoperative issues

To achieve a successful repair, preoperative studies must confirm the diagnosis and localize the site of the CSF leak. β_2-Transferrin is a protein present only in CSF, perilymph, and aqueous humor. Only 0.17 mL of nasal fluid is needed for testing using newer laboratory techniques [15], but this may be difficult to obtain in cases of intermittent leaks. False-positive and false-negative results are unlikely with β_2-transferrin testing, but can occur

[16]. β_2-Transferrin provides an accurate, noninvasive method to establish the diagnosis of an active CSF leak, but it provides little information on the precise location of the leak. Beta trace protein is another noninvasive marker that is specific for CSF and is used most commonly in Europe [17].

Preoperative imaging for endoscopic CSF leak repairs always requires coronal and, in some cases, axial CT scans to define the bony anatomy. If the diagnosis is in doubt or the patient is unable to collect fluid for β_2-transferrin, a CT cisternogram may be performed at the same time, but this requires a lumbar puncture. MRI may be useful, particularly in cases in which neoplasms or other intracranial pathology are present, but is not required in all cases [18,19]. Radioactive cisternograms are used less commonly today because they are less accurate in making a definitive diagnosis and localizing the site of the leak. Radioactive cisternograms may improve diagnostic sensitivity in cases of low volume or intermittent leaks because the pledgets remain in place for several hours.

Preoperative intrathecal fluorescein (as described subsequently in the surgical technique section) with a thorough endoscopic examination is useful in establishing the diagnosis of CSF leak, but its ability to localize the leak site precisely may be limited. If a patient has not had prior sinus surgery, skull base exposure is limited. If extensive sinus surgery was performed previously with adequate exposure of the skull base, it may be helpful and accurate. Most estimates place the accuracy around 96%, but there still can be false-positive and false-negative results. Intraoperatively, when wide surgical exposure is obtained, intrathecal fluorescein is useful in localizing the defect and ensuring a watertight closure. Depending on the rate of the leak, the rate of CSF turnover, and the timing of the intrathecal injection, the fluorescein may be significantly diluted or excreted by the time of surgery. Use of a blue light filter can improve the detection of dilute fluorescein.

Deciding which preoperative test is needed for a given patient should be based on the clinical picture and the precise information needed. The invasiveness of the diagnostic test and the risks to the patient also should be taken into account.

Intraoperative concerns

Lumbar drain and intrathecal fluorescein

In appropriate cases, a lumbar drain is placed before beginning the surgical approach. Patients with high-volume CSF leaks can have a relative depletion of CSF, and it can be difficult to identify the subarachnoid space and withdraw CSF or place the lumbar drain. In these cases, it may be easiest to place the lumbar drain with the patient awake and in a sitting position to fill the lumbar cistern with CSF. The other option is to place the lumbar drain after intubation and elevate the head of the bed to assist in dilating the lumbar cistern with CSF.

Fluorescein (0.1 mL of 10% solution diluted in 10 mL of CSF) is injected slowly into the intrathecal space through the spinal needle over 10 minutes. Fluorescein can aid in precise identification of the bony skull base defect and associated CSF leak. The authors have not noted any complications from fluorescein, when used as described. Complications usually are related to higher concentrations, more rapid injections, or suboccipital punctures [20]. After fluorescein instillation is complete, the lumbar catheter is inserted, secured, and clamped for the initial portion of the case. It may be difficult to inject fluorescein through the lumbar catheter; the authors prefer to inject it through the spinal needle before catheter insertion. Later in the surgical case, after the skull base defect is exposed, and preparations for graft placement are being made, 10 to 15 mL of CSF is removed over 15 minutes to aid in reduction of the cauterized encephalocele base. After graft placement, the lumbar drain is kept open and draining 5 to 10 mL per hour for the remainder of the procedure and for the initial postoperative period. Diligent care of the lumbar drain is required during the immediate postoperative period. The temptation to clamp the drain during patient extubation or transport should be resisted; this is precisely when the greatest risk exists for ICP elevation owing to coughing, Valsalva maneuvers, and patient movement that would be transmitted against the graft. The height of the drain is adjusted to keep the drainage between 5 and 10 mL of CSF per hour.

The lumbar drain is most important during the first 24 hours after surgery. During this period, it is especially useful in avoiding large spikes in ICP if the patient coughs or strains during extubation or transport or has nausea and vomiting during the immediate postoperative period. Keeping the drain in longer than 24 to 48 hours probably does not provide any significant advantage to the repair. The tensile strength of the repair probably increases little during the first week. Most of the structural support of the repair rests on any underlay graft placed in the epidural space and on intranasal packing compressing the extracranial fascia or mucosa graft against the recipient bed. For most repairs, the authors clamp the lumbar drain for 6 to 12 hours to ensure leak cessation, then remove it on postoperative day 1 or 2. If the patient leaks, the lumbar drain can be reopened for 2 to 3 days or returned to the operating room for surgical exploration.

Positive-pressure ventilation

Positive-pressure ventilation in patients with a CSF leak carries the risk of pneumocephalus. Fatal cases have been reported from patients blowing their nose [21] or after pneumotoscopy [22] in the presence of patent cranial fistulas. To decrease this risk, the anesthesiologist can perform rapid-sequence intubation and minimize masking the patient and using positive-pressure ventilation.

Antibiotics

The authors do not use long-term prophylactic antibiotics in patients recently diagnosed with CSF leaks, but do use perioperative antibiotics. During surgery, tissue grafts are placed through the contaminated or colonized nasal cavity to rest against brain tissue at the skull base defect and risk a central nervous system infection. The authors generally use intravenous ceftriaxone because of its CSF penetration. Trimethoprim/sulfamethoxazole and levofloxacin are other alternatives that afford a degree of blood-brain barrier penetration and can be helpful in patients with cephalosporin allergies. Additionally, the authors irrigate the sinonasal cavity with clindamycin solution during the procedure in an attempt to minimize bacterial contamination and seeding of graft material.

Surgical approach

The exact surgical approach used for CSF leak repair depends on proper identification of the site of the skull base defect. At times, the site of the leak may be obvious from the patient's history and imaging studies, but in many cases, the use of intrathecal fluorescein, as described earlier, is extremely useful.

Ethmoid roof, cribriform, central sphenoid, and perisellar regions

Generally, leaks in the cribriform plate and ethmoid roof are treated with a standard transnasal endoscopic approach. After decongestion with topical and injected vasoconstrictors, the nose is irrigated with clindamycin to decrease bacteria within the surgical field and reduce the potential for intracranial seeding. A complete endoscopic ethmoidectomy and maxillary antrostomy usually are needed to provide adequate exposure of the skull base defect and leak. Frontal sinusotomies, sphenoidotomies, and middle/superior turbinectomies are performed if additional exposure is needed. Sinuses adjacent to the CSF leak site may need to be opened to prevent postoperative obstruction secondary to scarring or packing. Frontal sinusotomies and sphenoidotomies often are required even though the leak may be in the ethmoid roof or cribriform. These procedures proactively prevent the formation of iatrogenic mucoceles in the surrounding sinuses and minimize "collateral damage."

Defects in the central sphenoid can be approached through the endoscopic transethmoid or direct parasagittal approaches and a wide sphenoidotomy. Alternatively, the posterior nasal septum and intersinus septum can be resected for additional exposure of the midline perisellar or clival regions. Defects located in the lateral recess of the sphenoid sinus are difficult to access by the midline transeptal or transethmoid approaches and may require an endoscopic transpterygoid approach [23]. After a total ethmoidectomy, wide sphenoidotomy and wide maxillary antrostomy are performed, the posterior wall of the maxillary sinus is removed, and the pterygopalatine fossa is entered. The internal maxillary artery and its branches are identified, moved inferiorly, or clipped and divided to expose the deeper areas of the pterygopalatine fossa. Cranial nerve V2, the vidian nerve, and the sphenopalatine ganglion are dissected free and preserved if possible. The anterior wall of the sphenoid sinus that has pneumatized the pterygoid plates is drilled or curetted away to gain access to the lateral recess of the sphenoid sinus.

Frontal sinus

Frontal sinus CSF leaks generally can be divided into three anatomic sites: (1) immediately adjacent to the frontal recess, (2) direct frontal recess involvement, and (3) located within the frontal sinus proper. Although most leaks are limited to one of these distinct sites, some defects encompass multiple anatomic areas. This anatomic classification of skull base defect sites is clinically relevant because it often determines the surgical approach needed for repair [24].

Skull base defects located in the anterior-most portion of the ethmoid roof just posterior to the frontal recess do not involve the frontal sinus or its outflow tract directly because of their proximity; the frontal recess must be opened surgically to avoid iatrogenic mucoceles. Defects that directly involve the frontal recess may require a combined above-and-below approach using endoscopic and open techniques because the superior extent of the defect may be difficult to reach endoscopically, and the inferior/posterior extension of the defect may be difficult to reach from an external approach. The final anatomic site for frontal sinus CSF leaks is within the frontal sinus proper involving the posterior table above the isthmus of the frontal recess. Endoscopic approaches continue to expand with improved equipment and experience; however, defects located superiorly or laterally within the frontal sinus still may require an osteoplastic flap with or without obliteration. Frontal trephination and an endoscopic modified Lothrop procedure are adjuvant techniques that can be useful for unique cases of leaks that are located in the frontal sinus proper or possibly with extension into the frontal recess itself. The specific approach depends on the site and size of the defect, the equipment available, and surgical experience.

Intracranial approach

Otorhinolaryngologists now are able to access all areas of the anterior and central skull base successfully, but there are still limitations to extracranial approaches. These may include multiple, comminuted defects, broadly attenuated or badly deformed skull bases, tumors with intracranial extension that are not amenable to endoscopic resection, large bilateral defects in an anosmic patient, and high-pressure leaks requiring CSF diversion procedures.

Preparation of recipient bed

When the skull base defect is localized, and adequate exposure has been obtained via an appropriate surgical approach, the recipient bed is prepared by removing several millimeters of mucosa surrounding the bony defect. Sinus mucosa continues to secrete mucus and may separate the graft from the recipient bed if it is not removed; it is crucial to remove the mucosa thoroughly to expose the underlying bone. The authors do not attempt to remove 100% of the mucosa within a given sinus, unless a defect located in the periphery of the frontal sinus is being treated, and it is planned to obliterate the frontal sinus. This approach is particularly applicable for sphenoid leaks, for which it is virtually impossible to remove all mucosa from the lateral aspects of the sphenoid. When appropriate mucosa is removed, a diamond burr or curette can be used to abrade the recipient bed bone lightly and stimulate osteoneogenesis.

When the borders of the bony skull base defect are prepared, any encephaloceles are reduced using bipolar cautery as much as possible. Malleable suction monopolar cautery devices can be used selectively within the ethmoid cavity and are particularly useful for reaching difficult areas in the anterior and lateral skull base. Monopolar cautery is avoided near or adjacent to the lamina papyracea, optic nerve, or carotid arteries.

As the encephalocele is progressively ablated, meticulous hemostasis is required. Hemostasis is especially important when treating the encephalocele base to avoid the potentially devastating complication of intracranial hemorrhage. This complication could occur if the encephalocele was sharply resected or avulsed and the base retracted intracranially. Precise application of electrocautery to the stalk or base helps prevent intracranial bleeding. When the encephalocele base is reduced, if a lumbar drain has been placed preoperatively, the drain is opened, and CSF is diverted away from the graft site and into the collection bag. Removing approximately 10 to 15 mL and positioning the collection bag to establish a flow rate of 5 to 10 mL/h allows the encephalocele base to be reduced intracranially, facilitating intracranial graft placement.

Skull base reconstruction

When an appropriate surgical approach with adequate exposure has been performed, and the recipient bed is prepared with ablation of any encephaloceles that may be present, skull base reconstruction is undertaken. The decision of how to reconstruct the skull base depends on the cause of the leak, the size of the resultant bony defect, and the underlying ICP [25]. Small defects of 2 to 3 mm or simple cracks in the skull base make it difficult to place an underlay graft within the epidural space, and in these cases, a simple soft tissue overlay graft suffices. Defects of moderate size (≥ 4 mm) and with normal underlying ICPs, such as after a tumor resection, can be reconstructed successfully in a multilayer fashion, using soft tissue for underlay and overlay grafts. Extremely large defects or smaller defects with elevated ICPs, such as spontaneous CSF leaks or leaks with hydrocephalus, probably benefit from a rigid underlay graft to provide structural support followed by a soft tissue overlay graft.

For underlay grafts, the repair is performed by gently elevating the dura above the bony skull base defect and placing grafts in the epidural space. An otologic elevator is helpful in dissecting the dura and defining the epidural space. When bone grafts are used, care in graft design and placement is needed. In some patients, such as patients with spontaneous leaks, the entire skull base is attenuated and can fracture easily, creating an even larger defect. These defects often have complex three-dimensional configurations, requiring precise shaping of the bone graft. Donor options are septal or mastoid bone. When the bone graft is of satisfactory size and shape, it is soaked in clindamycin solution to decrease the risk of intracranial seeding of bacteria. The graft is placed carefully in the epidural space to close the bony defect. We generally do not use cartilage grafts because of their increased thickness, tendency to fracture, and lower structural strength compared with bone grafts. When using soft tissue underlay grafts, the technique is identical. Although a variety of rigid and soft tissue grafts have been used successfully, it is imperative not to place mucosal grafts in an underlay fashion. Doing so may result in mucoceles, meningitis, or other central nervous system complications (Fig. 4).

After positioning an appropriate underlay graft (if needed), an overlay graft is placed over the entire repair. Care must be taken not to obstruct surrounding sinuses, leading to iatrogenic mucoceles. Multiple layers of absorbable packing follow the overlay graft. In certain locations, such as the sella or sphenoid sinus, abdominal fat may be used to augment or replace absorbable packing. In these cases, the fat serves as biologic packing and

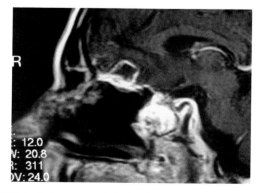

Fig. 4. Iatrogenic CSF leak that occurred during functional endoscopic sinus surgery was repaired using a middle turbinate graft (elsewhere). This patient had a seizure, and subsequent endoscopic re-exploration showed the mucosal covered graft approximately 2 cm intracranially. Note ring-enhancing lesion on sagittal T1-weighted MRI.

is not intended to obliterate the sphenoid completely, but rather to serve as temporary support with the goal of maintaining long-term patency of the sinus. In contrast to frontal sinus obliterations in which complete mucosal removal is possible via an osteoplastic approach, it is virtually impossible to remove all mucosa completely from the sphenoid.

Graft materials

Multiple varieties of grafting materials and placement techniques have been described, and most have been successful. The specific graft material chosen depends on the size and location of defect, the anatomic character of the defect and recipient bed, and the presence of elevated CSF pressure. Each skull base defect, meningoencephalocele, and leak is unique; an algorithmic approach is not optimal. Experimental evidence shows that a free graft guides wound healing by acting as a scaffold [26]. Free grafts are adherent to bone at 1 week and replaced by fibrous connective tissue at 3 weeks with some degree of postoperative contracture. We generally recommend a multilayer closure, when possible, that includes an underlay graft placed in the epidural space followed by an overlay graft placed intranasally against exposed bone around the defect. This type of repair provides structural support from the underlay graft in the epidural space and watertight closure from the overlay graft.

Soft tissue grafts can be autologous temporalis fascia, alloplastic collagen materials (eg, Duragen), cadaveric fascia, pericardium, or dermis. All of these materials have the advantage of being readily available and acceptable for either underlay or overlay grafts. None has shown superior efficacy, and choice depends on the surgeon's preference. Alternatively, numerous authors use free mucosal grafts for soft tissue reconstruction. Septal and inferior turbinate mucosae are relatively thick and provide sufficient graft material for most repairs. Middle turbinate mucosa also is an option, but it tends to be thinner, and there is less material available. Composite grafts using turbinate bone and mucosa provide a two-layer closure, but both layers are placed simultaneously in an overlay fashion and do not have the stability of an epidural graft. In addition, it is difficult to sculpt the bony portion of a composite graft to fit the skull base defect precisely while it is still attached to its mucosal covering. As previously mentioned, the reader is cautioned that mucosal soft tissue grafts must be placed so that the mucosal surface is oriented into the sinonasal cavity. Placement of mucosa in the epidural space or reversing its orientation can lead to intracranial mucoceles, meningitis, or other central nervous system complications.

Tissue adhesives

A variety of tissue adhesives have been reported anecdotally for CSF leak repairs, but no scientific clinical studies have been conducted. One experimental study using a mouse model showed an apparent advantage to using fibrin sealant with a free muscle graft [27]. If tissue adhesives are used, they must be applied conservatively because a thick layer of adhesive may prevent the graft material from coming into contact with the wound bed.

Packing

Degradable packing materials, such as Gelfoam, Surgicel, and Avitene, have been used with success. There is no proven scientific advantage to any one product. Gelfilm or Silastic sheeting used between multiple layers of packing may prevent the inadvertent removal or movement of all the layers of packing and possible disruption of the graft during the early postoperative period.

Postoperative issues

Activity

All patients are kept at strict bed rest while lumbar drains are in place. After the lumbar drain is removed, patients gradually resume ambulation. Patients are instructed on movement techniques to avoid breath holding and Valsalva maneuvers and are encouraged to inhale or exhale continuously when changing position. The authors encourage light activity for 6 weeks after surgery.

Bed position and lumbar drain management

Alterations in bed position alter the CSF pressure at the graft site. When the patient is lying perfectly flat, the ICP is roughly equivalent at all points from the lumbar cistern to the skull base. As the head of bed is raised, CSF pressure at the anterior skull base decreases, while the pressure in the lumbar cistern increases proportionally. Brain parenchyma also may help to maintain the position of epidural grafts when the patient is raised to the sitting position. The authors keep patients slightly elevated at 15° while the lumbar drain is in place. In patients with suspected ICP elevation, additional clinical information that may be important for future management decisions can be obtained by measuring ICPs through the lumbar drain as described elsewhere [13]. When the drain is removed, the authors allow approximately 4 hours for the lumbar drain catheter site to seal. Thereafter, the authors gradually elevate the head of the bed to 30° to decrease the CSF pressure at the skull base defect repair site. If patients do well and do not exhibit any signs of a spinal headache, they can be advanced to a sitting position and light activity.

Acetazolamide

Acetazolamide (Diamox) is a diuretic that can decrease CSF production 48% [28]. The authors have begun to use it in cases in which elevated ICP plays a role. Acetazolamide has reduced ICP in several spontaneous leak patients and improved their symptoms of pulsatile tinnitus and pressure-type headaches. The optimal timing, dosing, and long-term benefits of this approach have not been proven, but it may reduce the risk of developing subsequent skull base defects in patients with elevated CSF pressures. The authors periodically monitor electrolytes in any patient placed on long-term diuretic therapy.

Endoscopic care

Patients are seen every 1 to 2 weeks postoperatively. Conservative endoscopic débridement is performed to maintain patency of the dependent sinuses surrounding the repair to avoid stasis of secretions and bacterial infections. The area of the packing and graft specifically are avoided to allow adequate healing. By 6 weeks postoperatively, most patients have returned to relatively normal activity levels, and little packing remains.

Continuous positive airway pressure

The authors have repaired several patients with obstructive sleep apnea who use continuous positive airway pressure. The authors restrict the use of continuous positive airway pressure during the immediate postoperative period, to avoid the risk of pneumocephalus from positive-pressure ventilation. All of the authors' patients have been able to resume using continuous positive airway pressure safely 4 to 6 weeks after surgery.

Summary

The role of the otolaryngologist in diagnosing and treating CSF leaks of the anterior and central skull base continues to expand. A comprehensive understanding of the physiology, pathology, diagnosis, and treatment approaches is crucial to treat this wide variety of skull base defects properly.

References

[1] Lanza DC, O'Brien DA, Kennedy DW. Endoscopic repair of cerebrospinal fluid fistulae and encephaloceles. Laryngoscope 1996;106:1119–25.
[2] Mattox DE, Kennedy DW. Endoscopic management of cerebrospinal fluid leaks and cephaloceles. Laryngoscope 1990;100:857–62.
[3] Daube JR, Reagan TJ, Sandok BA, et al. The cerebrospinal fluid system. In: Daube JR, Reagan TJ, Sandok BA, et al, editors. Medical neurosciences: an approach to anatomy, pathology, and physiology by systems and levels. 2nd edition. Boston: Little, Brown; 1986. p. 93–111.
[4] Zlab MK, Moore GF, Daly DT, et al. Cerebrospinal fluid rhinorrhea: a review of the literature. Ear Nose Throat J 1992;71:314–7.
[5] Bernal-Sprekelsen M, Bleda-Vazquez C, Carrau RL. Ascending meningitis secondary to traumatic cerebrospinal fluid leaks. Am J Rhinol 2000;14:257–9.

[6] Gassner HG, Ponikau JU, Sherris DA, Kern EB. CSF rhinorrhea: 95 consecutive surgical cases with long term follow-up at the Mayo Clinic. Am J Rhinol 1999;13:439–47.

[7] Woodworth BA, Schlosser RJ, Faust RA, Bolger WE. Evolutions in management of congenital intranasal skull base defects. Arch Otolaryngol Head Neck Surg 2004;130:1283–8.

[8] Woodworth BA, Schlosser RJ. Endoscopic repair of a congenital nasal encephalocele in a 23 month old infant. Int J Pediatr Otorhinolaryngol 2005;69:1007–9.

[9] Hubbard JL, McDonald TJ, Pearson BW, Laws ER Jr. Spontaneous cerebrospinal fluid rhinorrhea: evolving concepts in diagnosis and surgical management based on the Mayo Clinic experience from 1970 through 1981. Neurosurgery 1985;16:314–21.

[10] Ommaya AK, Di Chiro G, Baldwin M, Pennybacker JB. Non-traumatic cerebrospinal fluid rhinorrhea. J Neurol Neurosurg Psychiatry 1968;31:214–25.

[11] Schlosser RJ, Bolger WE. Management of multiple spontaneous nasal meningoencephaloceles. Laryngoscope 2002;112:980–5.

[12] Schlosser RJ, Bolger WE. Significance of empty sella in cerebrospinal fluid leaks. Otolaryngol Head Neck Surg 2003;128:32–8.

[13] Schlosser RJ, Wilensky EM, Grady MS, Bolger WE. Elevated intracranial pressures in spontaneous CSF leaks. Am J Rhinol 2003;17:191–5.

[14] Schick B, Ibing R, Brors D, Draf W. Long-term study of endonasal duraplasty and review of the literature. Ann Otol Rhinol Laryngol 2001;110:142–7.

[15] Papadea C, Schlosser RJ. Sensitive detection of beta-2 transferrin in cerebrospinal fluid leakage using an automated immunofixation electrophoresis method. Clin Chem 2004;51: 464–70.

[16] Skedros DG, Cass SP, Hirsch BE, Kelly RH. Sources of error in use of beta-2 transferrin analysis for diagnosing perilymphatic and cerebral spinal fluid leaks. Otolaryngol Head Neck Surg 1993;109:861–4.

[17] Arrer E, Meco C, Oberascher G, et al. Beta trace protein as a marker for cerebrospinal fluid rhinorrhea. Clin Chem 2002;48:939–41.

[18] Stone JA, Castillo M, Neelon B, Mukherji SK. Evaluation of CSF leaks: high resolution CT compared with contrast-enhanced CT and radionuclide cisternography. AJNR Am J Neuroradiol 1999;20:706–12.

[19] Shetty PG, Shroff MM, Sahani DV, Kirtane MV. Evaluation of high-resolution CT and MR cisternography in the diagnosis of cerebrospinal fluid fistula. AJNR Am J Neuroradiol 1998; 19:633–9.

[20] Wolf G, Greistorfer K, Stammberger H. Endoscopic detection of cerebrospinal fluid fistulas with a fluorescence technique: report of experiences with over 925 cases. Laryngorhinootologie 1997;76:588–94.

[21] Komisar A, Weitz S, Ruben RJ. Rhinorrhea and pneumocephalus after cerebrospinal fluid shunting. Otolaryngol Head Neck Surg 1986;94:194–7.

[22] Finsnes KA. Lethal intracranial complication following air insufflation with a pneumatic otoscope. Acta Otolaryngol 1973;75:436–8.

[23] Bolger WE, Osenbach R. Endoscopic transpterygoid approach to the lateral sphenoid recess. Ear Nose Throat J 1999;78:36–46.

[24] Woodworth BA, Schlosser RJ. Frontal sinus CSF leaks. In: Draf W, Senior B, Kountakis S, editors. The frontal sinus. Heidelberg, Germany: Springer; 2005. p. 143–52.

[25] Schlosser RJ, Bolger WE. Nasal cerebrospinal fluid leaks: critical review and surgical considerations. Laryngoscope 2004;114:255–65.

[26] Gjuric M, Goede U, Keimer H, Wigand ME. Endonasal endoscopic closure of cerebrospinal fluid fistulas at the anterior cranial base. Ann Otol Rhinol Laryngol 1996;105:620–3.

[27] Nishihira S, McCaffrey TV. The use of fibrin glue for the repair of experimental CSF rhinorrhea. Laryngoscope 1988;98:625–7.

[28] Carrion E, Hertzog JH, Medlock MD, et al. Use of acetazolamide to decrease cerebrospinal fluid production in chronically ventilated patients with ventriculopleural shunts. Arch Dis Child 2001;84:68–71.

ELSEVIER
SAUNDERS

Otolaryngol Clin N Am
39 (2006) 539–549

OTOLARYNGOLOGIC
CLINICS
OF NORTH AMERICA

Powered Endoscopic Dacryocystorhinostomy

P.J. Wormald, MD, FRACS, FCS (SA), FRCS, MBChB

Department of Surgery–Otolaryngology, Head and Neck Surgery,
Adelaide and Flinders Universities, The Queen Elizabeth Hospital, 28 Woodville Road,
Woodville, South Australia 5011, Australia

Over the past 10 years the interest in endoscopic dacryocystorhinostomy (DCR) has increased with improved instruments and endoscopic sinus surgery skills. Although endoscopic DCR was first described in 1989 [1], the technique has evolved over the past 15 years as the understanding of the anatomy [2] and ability to achieve reliable and consistent results has improved [3–6].

Assessment of nasolacrimal duct obstruction

The patient presenting with epiphora is evaluated clinically to ensure that other causes of epiphora, such as lid malposition, entropion, ectropion, punctal abnormalities, and inflammatory causes such as blepharitis, have been excluded. The medial canthal region is palpated for a mucocele. Pressure is placed on the medial canthal region and the puncta inspected for reflux of mucous or purulent material, which would indicate obstruction of the nasolacrimal system. The inferior or superior punctum is dilated and a Bowman's lacrimal probe is gently slid along the canaliculus toward the lacrimal sac. A hard stop normally means that the probe entered the sac and stopped on the medial bony wall of the sac. A soft stop means that the probe stopped at the entrance to the sac, which may either indicate a tight common canaliculus sac junction or a stenosis of the common canaliculus. The patency of the nasolacrimal system is assessed by syringing. A blunt lacrimal needle (25-gauge) is introduced into the inferior punctum

---

P.J. Wormald receives royalties for the design of instruments from Medtronic Xomed.
E-mail address: peterj.wormald@adelaide.edu.au

and saline is injected. If the lacrimal system is obstructed, reflux of saline will occur through the upper punctum. If saline passes into the nose without reflux, the lacrimal system is patent. Clinicians should remember that syringing generates abnormal pressures in the lacrimal system and the ability for saline to penetrate into the nose may not reflect an underlying symptomatic narrowing of the nasolacrimal system.

Depending on the patency of the nasolacrimal system, obstruction can be either anatomic or functional [6]. Anatomic obstruction occurs when the nasolacrimal system is obstructed, usually between the lacrimal sac and nasal cavity, and is indicated by reflux on syringing and impeded flow of radioopaque dye during a dacryocystogram (DCG) (Fig. 1). Functional obstruction is less common (± 30%) and is believed to be a narrowing of the nasolacrimal apparatus, a failure of the lacrimal pump system, or a combination of the two [6]. Functional obstruction is diagnosed when the nasolacrimal system is patent on syringing and DCG (Fig. 2A). In these patients, function of the lacrimal system is assessed using a lacrimal scintillogram. A radioisotope is placed in the conjunctiva and the progress of this isotope through the nasolacrimal system is monitored for 30 minutes. Inability to penetrate the nasal cavity indicates a functional nasolacrimal obstruction (Fig. 2B) [6]. The scintillogram can provide further diagnostic information by identifying if the isotope collects in the lacrimal sac. If isotope collection is seen, then the cause is less likely to be a failure of the lacrimal pump than a narrowing in the nasolacrimal system that is preventing the normal progression of tears into the nose, and a DCR should be beneficial. As shown in the "Results" section, the diagnosis of either an anatomic or functional obstruction affects the prognosis of the DCR [6]. This ability to define the type of nasolacrimal obstruction allows the patient to be informed of the prognosis and have realistic expectations about what can be achieved through surgery.

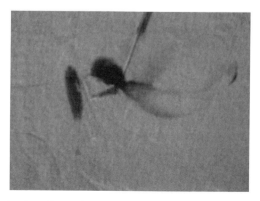

Fig. 1. Left DCG showing obstruction of the nasolacrimal duct with reflux of contrast into conjunctiva.

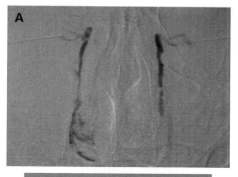

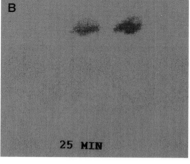

Fig. 2. (*A*) Bilateral DCGs illustrating patency of the nasolacrimal system bilaterally with penetration of contrast into the nasal cavity. (*B*) Bilateral lacrimal scintillography showing bilateral obstruction of tear flow with no nasal penetration of isotope at 25 minutes into the nasal cavity.

Development of endoscopic dacryocystorhinostomy

In the early 1990s, endoscopic DCR was performed by identifying the frontal process of the maxilla–lacrimal bone junction and then removing the frontal process of the maxilla superiorly with a rongeur up to the level of the insertion of the middle turbinate onto the lateral nasal wall (the so-called "axilla" of the middle turbinate) [7]. In most cases the bone became progressively thicker as the dissection proceeded up the lateral nasal wall and the dissection had to stop (because the surgeon was unable to engage the rongeur) well short of the axilla of the middle turbinate. The success of this technique was in the low 80% [6], causing some criticism of the technique by the oculoplastic surgeons who were able to achieve results in the low 90% [8]. The major difference between the techniques seemed to be that the oculoplastic surgeons achieved complete exposure of the lacrimal sac and then achieved lacrimal mucosa to nasal mucosa apposition through suturing the lacrimal and nasal mucosa [3]. To achieve complete exposure of the lacrimal sac, a better understanding of the intranasal siting of the lacrimal sac was necessary. We conducted a study in which we filled the lacrimal sac with radio-opaque dye and performed CT scans of the lacrimal apparatus and nasal cavity [2]. This procedure allowed accurate definition of the position of the lacrimal sac relative to the axilla of the middle turbinate. This study placed the major portion of the lacrimal sac above the axilla of the middle turbinate rather than anteroinferior to the axilla as was previously believed (Fig. 3).

This knowledge has allowed us to develop a new surgical technique that has imitated the external DCR procedure by allowing exposure of the entire lacrimal sac during endoscopic dissection, thereby allowing creation of the biggest possible opening in the lacrimal sac [3–5]. The creation of the largest possible ostium minimizes the risk for subsequent stenosis and closure of the lacrimal ostium [9]. The technique described later also imitates the external procedure in that the lacrimal and nasal mucosa are closely approximated, allowing first-intention healing rather than second-intention (granulation tissue) healing [3]. The absence of postoperative granulation tissue lessens the risk for subsequent fibrosis, stenosis, and closure of the ostium.

Surgical technique

Surgical technique [3–5] begins with assessment of the nasal septum. Any significant deflection of the septum in the region of the axilla of the middle turbinate should be handled with a limited septoplasty and resection of the cartilage or bone in this region. When the surgeon creates the space to operate, the risks for poor surgical technique with limited exposure of the sac and for postoperative adhesion formation between the septum and the lateral nasal wall are minimized. After the nose has been decongested, the lateral nasal wall is infiltrated with 2% lidocaine and 1:80:000 adrenaline above and anterior to the axilla. A 30° endoscope is preferred for this procedure

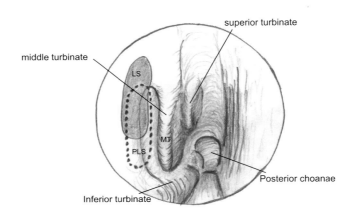

Fig. 3. Endoscopic view into the right nasal cavity showing the previous incorrect lacrimal sac (PLS) position (outlined with a broken line) and the correct lacrimal sac (LS) position (shaded) above and anterior to the middle turbinate (MT).

because most of the surgery occurs on the lateral nasal wall and the angulation of the endoscope allows improved visualization of the lateral wall. During surgery the 30° endoscope is always held above the surgical site looking directly laterally with all instruments passed below the endoscope.

A #15 scalpel blade is used to make the superior horizontal mucosal incision starting 3 to 5 mm posterior to and about 8 to 10 mm above the axilla of the middle turbinate (Fig. 4). This incision is brought 10 mm anterior to the axilla onto the frontal process of the maxilla. The incision is turned vertically and brought inferiorly toward the insertion of the inferior turbinate. If measured against the middle turbinate, this incision extends about two thirds of the length of the anterior end of the middle turbinate. Just above the insertion of the inferior turbinate on the lateral nasal wall the scalpel is turned horizontally and the incision continued posteriorly under the middle turbinate up to the insertion of the uncinate. The placement of this mucosal incision is crucial to the success of the procedure; an incision that is placed too low will not allow full exposure of the sac and an incision that is not brought far enough anteriorly will result in a short flap that will get sucked into the drill during removal of the bone over the sac.

Once the incision has been made, a suction Freer elevator is used to raise the flap (Fig. 5). When the flap is raised and the bone falls away, care should be taken to keep the tip of the elevator on the bone as the dissection proceeds over the prominence of the maxilla's frontal process to its junction with the thin lacrimal bone. This junction must be identified because it provides a critical landmark for removal of the maxilla's frontal process and subsequent identification of the lacrimal sac (Fig. 5). This junction is best identified just above the insertion of the inferior turbinate because the lacrimal bone ends about 5 mm below the axilla.

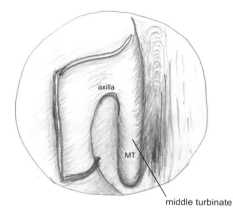

Fig. 4. Incisions for raising mucosal flap starting 8 to 10 mm above axilla of middle turbinate (MT) and coming 10 mm anterior to the axilla.

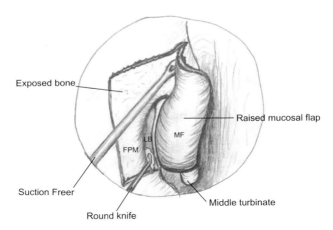

Fig. 5. Elevation of the mucosal flap (MF) by a suction Freer. The hard bone of the frontal process of the maxilla (FPM) and its junction with the lacrimal bone (LB) are clearly identified before the round knife is used to remove the lacrimal bone from the posterior inferior portion of the lacrimal sac.

A round knife (from the ear instrument set) is used to fracture the thin lacrimal bone and remove as much of it as possible (Fig. 5). This procedure allows introduction of the Hajek-Koeffler punch and engagement and removal of the free edge of the frontal process of the maxilla (Fig. 6). This bone removal is continued as far superiorly as possible until the bone becomes too thick for the punch to engage the bone. However, this bone removal usually finishes well short of the axilla of the middle turbinate. To

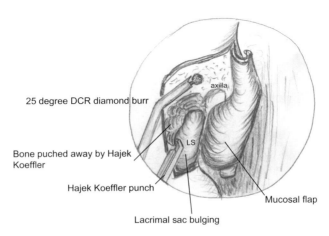

Fig. 6. The rongeur is used to remove as much of the frontal process of the maxilla as possible before the curved DCR diamond burr is used to expose the remaining lacrimal sac (LS) and agger nasi cell above the axilla of the middle turbinate.

avoid pinching the wall of the sac and tearing the sac with the rongeurs, the jaws should be opened after each bite, allowing any sac wall that may have become caught to be released before the bone is removed. The powered endoscopic microdebrider with a Rough Diamond 2.5-mm DCR Burr (Medtronic Xomed, Jacksonville, Florida) is used to first thin down the remaining bone and then to remove it by following the sac superiorly until the edge of the superior mucosal incision is reached (Fig. 6). Care must be taken to ensure that the burr does not slip under the bone edge adjacent to the sac mucosa during this dissection because the mucosa of the sac is thin and prolonged contact with the burr will result in a hole in the sac wall. As the posterosuperior bone is removed, the mucosa from the agger nasi cell is seen (Fig. 7). In most cases the agger nasi cell will be exposed as the superior sac is exposed.

Once the sac has been completely exposed, the inferior or superior punctum is dilated and the lacrimal sac cannulated with a lacrimal probe. The tip of the probe must be clearly visualized behind the very thin lacrimal sac wall. Often the sac wall will move with the probe placed at the common canaliculus entry to the sac and the probe will appear to be in the sac. The surgeon must not make an incision into the sac wall until the tip is clearly seen because this could result in damage to the common canaliculus opening as the incision is made onto the tip of the probe. Once the tip of the probe is clearly seen tenting the medial sac wall, the Lacrimal Spear Knife (Medtronic Xomed, Jacksonville Florida) is used to make a vertical incision into the sac wall (Fig. 7). The sac is opened from top to bottom and the lacrimal probe should be seen coming through the common canaliculus opening. The lacrimal mini-sickle knife is used to make a releasing incision at the top of the vertical incision and at the bottom of the incision, which should

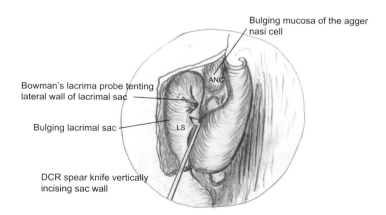

Bulging mucosa of the agger nasi cell

Bowman's lacrima probe tenting lateral wall of lacrimal sac

ANC

Bulging lacrimal sac

LS

DCR spear knife vertically incising sac wall

Fig. 7. A Bowman's lacrimal probe is placed into the lacrimal sac and the medial wall of the lacrimal sac (LS) is tented. A DCR spear knife is used to incise the sac vertically from top to bottom. The exposed mucosa of the agger nasi cell (ANC) is visible above the axilla.

allow the anterior lacrimal flap to be rolled out and remain flat on the lateral nasal wall (Fig. 8). The soft tissue scissors are used to make similar cuts in the posterior flap, allowing the posterior flap to be rolled out until it is also flat against the lateral nasal wall. The mucosa of the agger nasi cell is opened vertically and the edge of this mucosa approximated to the posterior superior lacrimal mucosa. The original nasal mucosal flap is trimmed so that this flap mucosa approximates the lacrimal mucosa along the superior, posterior, and inferior edges of the opened lacrimal sac (Fig. 9). This approximation allows the lacrimal sac and nasal mucosa edges to heal through primary intention and lessens the amount of granulation tissue that forms, thereby lessening the risk for scar tissue formation and procedure failure.

Silastic O'Donaghue tubes (B.D. Visitec, Bidford-Upon-Avon, UK) are placed through the upper and lower canaliculus and brought out of the common canaliculus. These tubes are placed to dilate the common canaliculus opening into the lacrimal sac, which is important especially in patients who have functional (ie, a patent system on DCG but with impaired nasal penetration on lacrimal scintilography) epiphora. As the lacrimal sac is widely marsupialized into the nasal cavity, these tubes are placed specifically to dilate the common canaliculus entry into the lacrimal sac rather than to keep the sac open. A 4-mm diameter, 1-cm long piece of Silastic tubing is slid over the Silastic tubes as a spacer. A loop of Silastic tubing is pulled in the medial canthus region to ensure that no tension is placed on the tubing (Fig. 10). Tension on the Silastic tubing can cause the tubing to cut through the puncta, resulting in a loss of function. A 1.5 × 1.5-cm piece of Gelfoam (Pharmacia & Uphjohn Company, Kalamazoo, Michigan) is placed over the tubes and slid into position to hold the flaps in place. Ligar clips are placed just below the spacer and the Silastic tubes cut. The Gelfoam is lifted and the position of the flaps checked before the Gelfoam is replaced.

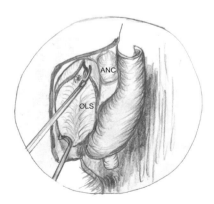

Fig. 8. To allow the lacrimal sac mucosal flaps to be rolled out to fully open the lacrimal sac (OLS), a DCR mini-sickle knife is used to make anterior releasing incisions inferiorly and superiorly and the soft tissue scissors is used to make posterior releasing incisions superiorly and inferiorly. ANC, agger nasi cell.

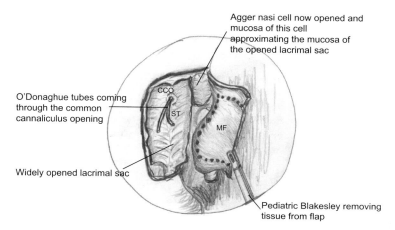

Agger nasi cell now opened and
mucosa of this cell
approximating the mucosa of
the opened lacrimal sac

O'Donaghue tubes coming
through the common
cannaliculus opening

CCO

ST

MF

Widely opened lacrimal sac

Pediatric Blakesley removing
tissue from flap

Fig. 9. After the lacrimal sac has been fully opened and the agger nasi cell has been opened, inferior and superior mucosal flaps are created by removing the tissue within the broken line of the mucosal flap (MF) using a pediatric Blakesley forceps. The Silastic tubes (ST) are placed through the common canaliculus opening (CCO), which is clearly visible in the lateral wall of the lacrimal sac.

The patient is given broad-spectrum antibiotics for 5 days and Chloromycetin eye drops for 10 days. Saline nasal douches are started postoperatively. The O'Donaghue tubes are removed at 4 weeks.

Results

When reporting results, *success* must be defined accurately [3–6,10]. In our published studies [3–6,10], a successful DCR was defined as a patient

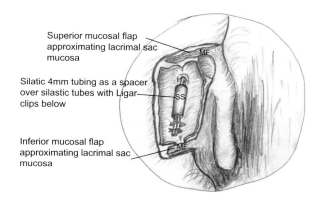

Superior mucosal flap
approximating lacrimal sac
mucosa

MF

Silatic 4mm tubing as a spacer
over silastic tubes with Ligar
clips below

SS

Inferior mucosal flap
approximating lacrimal sac
mucosa

MF

Fig. 10. The superior and inferior mucosal flaps (MF) are placed over the raw bone ensuring mucosa-to-mucosa apposition. Note the posterior superior lacrimal mucosa is apposed to the opened agger nasi cell mucosa. A Silastic spacer (SS) is placed over the Silastic tubes and Ligar clips applied below the spacer.

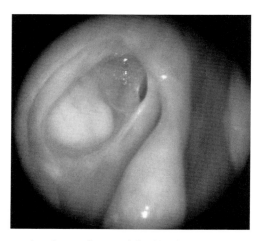

Fig. 11. Right postoperative picture of marsupialized lacrimal sac. Note bubbles from common canaliculus opening.

who is asymptomatic and has a healed patent lacrimal ostium with a free flow of fluorescein from the conjunctiva to the nose. Fig. 11 shows a typical result with a complete marsupialization of the right lacrimal sac into the nasal wall. The results with powered endoscopic DCR have been consistently successful for functional and anatomic obstruction in approximately 95% of patients [3–6,10]. Separating the results into anatomic versus functional obstruction, the success rate for anatomic obstruction is 97% but drops to 84% for functional obstruction [6]. Although 84% may seem low, most of the patients (>80%) in whom treatment was considered to have failed because they experienced ongoing symptoms, underwent a technically successful operation. These patients also form a small proportion of the total number of powered endoscopic DCRs, thereby decreasing the average success rate of all DCRs to 95% [3–6]. In this functional group, these patients (those who experienced treatment failure) still had symptoms, but most claimed these symptoms were much improved after the surgery. This technique has also been very effective in revision and pediatric DCR [10].

Summary

Powered endoscopic DCR is a reliable and effective technique for managing primary nasolacrimal duct obstruction in adults and children and for revision DCR.

References

[1] McDonogh M. Endoscopic transnasal dacryocystorhinostomy. Results in 21 patients. S Afr J Surg 1992;30:107–10.

[2] Wormald PJ, Kew J, van Hasselt CA. The intranasal anatomy of the naso-lacrimal sac in endoscopic dacryocystorhinostomy. Otolaryngol Head Neck Surg 2000;123:307–10.

[3] Wormald PJ. Powered endonasal dacryocystorhinostomy. Laryngoscope 2002;112:69–71.

[4] Tsirbas A, Wormald PJ. Endonasal dacryocystorhinostomy with mucosal flaps. Am J Ophthalmology 2003;135(1):76–83.

[5] Tsirbas A, Wormald PJ. Mechanical endonasal dacryocystorhinostomy versus external dacryocystorhinostomy. Ophthal Plast Reconstr Surg 2004;20(1):50–6.

[6] Wormald PJ, Tsirbas A. Investigation and endoscopic treatment for functional and anatomical obstruction of the nasolacrimal duct system. Clin Otolaryngol Allied Sci 2004;29(4): 352–6.

[7] Wormald PJ, Nilssen E. Endoscopic DCR: the team approach. Hong Kong Journal of Ophthalmology 1998;1:71–4.

[8] Hartikainen J, Antila J, Varpula M, et al. Prospective randomised comparison of endonasal endoscopic dacryocystorhinostomy and external dacryocystorhinostomy. Laryngoscope 1998;108:1861–6.

[9] Welham R, Wulc A. Management of unsuccessful lacrimal surgery. Br J Ophthalmol 1987; 71:152–7.

[10] Tsirbas A, Davis G, Wormald P. Revision DCR: a comparison of endoscopic and external techniques. Am J Rhinol 2005;19(3):322–5.

ELSEVIER
SAUNDERS

Otolaryngol Clin N Am
39 (2006) 551–561

OTOLARYNGOLOGIC
CLINICS
OF NORTH AMERICA

Endoscopic Orbital and Optic Nerve Decompression

Ralph Metson, MD[a,b,*], Steven D. Pletcher, MD[b]

[a]Department of Otology and Laryngology, Harvard Medical School, Boston, MA 02114, USA
[b]Department of Otolaryngology, Massachusetts Eye and Ear Infirmary,
243 Charles Street, Boston, MA 02114, USA

Soon after its introduction by Walsh and Ogura in the 1950s [1], transantral decompression of the orbit became a popular technique to treat patients with severe proptosis from Graves' disease. This procedure enabled otolaryngologists to remove the orbital floor and medial wall through the familiar Caldwell-Luc approach, allowing for decompression of the enlarged orbital muscles and fat into the maxillary and ethmoid sinuses. Soon after the introduction of endoscopic instrumentation for the performance of sinus surgery in the mid-1980s, however, surgeons began to experiment with an entirely transnasal approach to treat diseases of the orbit.

Kennedy et al [1] and Michel et al [2] first described endoscopic orbital decompression in the early 1990s. Because high-resolution endoscopes provided improved visualization in key anatomic regions, including the medial orbital wall and skull base, this technique soon gained widespread acceptance for the treatment of patients with Graves' disease, largely replacing the transantral approach. In addition to providing enhanced visualization, endoscopic instrumentation allowed for complete and safe bone removal, particularly along the orbital apex and optic canal. Although the use of endoscopic orbital decompression for the orbital manifestations of Graves' disease has been well established, the indications and applications for optic nerve decompression remain in evolution.

Graves' orbitopathy (dysthyroid orbitopathy)

Graves' disease is an autoimmune disorder that primarily affects the thyroid and the orbit. Thyroid manifestations are characterized by the

---

* Corresponding author. Zero Emerson Place, Suite 2D, Boston, MA 02114, USA.
  E-mail address: ralph_metson@meei.harvard.edu (R. Metson).

0030-6665/06/$ - see front matter © 2006 Elsevier Inc. All rights reserved.
doi:10.1016/j.otc.2006.01.004

production of autoantibodies to the thyrotropin receptor and subsequent hyperstimulation with resultant hyperthyroidism. The thyroid manifestations of Graves' disease generally are treated with medications, radiation (iodine 131), or surgery.

The orbital manifestations, known as dysthyroid orbitopathy, also represent an autoimmune process, although the exact antibody target is unclear. Inflammation with infiltration of T cells and increased glycosaminoglycan deposition results in enlargement of orbital fat and extraocular muscles. The increased orbital contents result in increased pressure within the bony orbit and resultant proptosis, compression of the optic nerve, or both. The degree of proptosis does not correlate with the overall severity of disease because patients with poor compliance of the orbital septum may not experience significant proptosis, but can have severe compression at the orbital apex and optic neuropathy. The orbital and thyroid manifestations of Graves' disease follow distinct and independent clinical courses.

Clinical manifestations of dysthyroid orbitopathy range from mild findings, such as tearing, photophobia, and conjunctival injection, to significant proptosis, diplopia, exposure keratopathy, and visual loss from optic neuropathy. The clinical course of Graves' orbitopathy can be divided into acute and chronic phases, with the acute phase characterized by active inflammation and lasting 6 to 18 months. The chronic phase is characterized by fibrosis and represents the preferred phase for surgical intervention.

Medical treatment of dysthyroid orbitopathy

Local measures, such as lubrication, eyelid taping, and patching, for patients with dryness and diplopia represent initial conservative treatment approaches. More aggressive treatments include the use of orbital radiation and systemic corticosteroids. Both treatments seem to be most effective during the acute phase of the disease. The use of orbital radiation is controversial, and its efficacy has been challenged by two more recent randomized prospective trials [3,4]. Systemic corticosteroid treatment shows symptomatic improvement, but symptoms generally recur after steroid treatment. Because of the deleterious side effects of long-term corticosteroid use, steroid treatment often is used as a temporizing measure or in conjunction with surgical decompression.

Endoscopic orbital decompression

The endoscopic technique allows for unmatched visualization of critical anatomic regions, such as the skull base and orbital apex, and avoids external or sublabial incisions. The entire medial orbital wall and the medial portion of the orbital floor is removed with endoscopic decompression (Fig. 1).

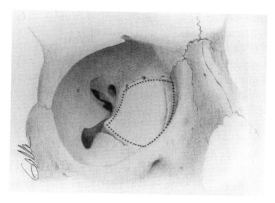

Fig. 1. Bone removed during endoscopic orbital decompression includes the entire medial wall of the orbit and the medial portion of the orbital floor with the lateral limit of decompression at the infraorbital nerve.

Technique

The patient is positioned in the supine position, and topical vasoconstriction is achieved with 4% cocaine pledgets. Draping is the same as with standard endoscopic sinus procedures, and the eyes are exposed in the surgical field, but protected with scleral shields. Image guidance systems may be used at the surgeon's discretion. Lidocaine 1% with 1:100,000 epinephrine is injected along the lateral nasal wall in the region of the maxillary line (a bony eminence that extends from the anterior attachment of the middle turbinate to the root of the inferior turbinate).

Surgery begins with an incision just posterior to the maxillary line and through the uncinate process. The uncinate process is medialized and removed; this allows visualization of the natural ostium of the maxillary sinus. With orbital decompression, it is necessary to open the maxillary sinus widely to achieve good access to the orbital floor and prevent blockage of the ostium from orbital fat, which protrudes after decompression. The ostium can be opened to the floor of the orbit superiorly, the wall of the maxillary sinus posteriorly, the thick bone of the frontal process of the maxilla anteriorly, and the inferior turbinate inferiorly. If the antrostomy is extended beyond the frontal process of the maxilla anteriorly, there is risk of damage to the nasolacrimal duct. Using a 30° endoscope, the wide antrostomy should allow easy visualization of the infraorbital nerve as it courses along the floor of the orbit.

An endoscopic sphenoethmoidectomy is performed in the standard fashion. After sphenoethmoidectomy, the anterior and posterior ethmoid arteries can be identified as they course along the skull base. We advocate removal of the middle turbinate during orbital decompression to optimize exposure of the medial orbital wall and facilitate postoperative cleanings.

An image guidance system may be used at this point to confirm removal of all ethmoid cells along the medial orbital wall.

When complete exposure of the medial orbital wall is obtained, a spoon curet is used to penetrate the thin bone of the lamina papyracea carefully (Fig. 2). This bone is elevated while preserving the underlying periorbita. Bone removal proceeds superiorly toward the ethmoid roof, inferiorly to the orbital floor, and anteriorly to the maxillary line. Bone in the region of the frontal recess is left intact; if bone is removed from this region, herniated fat may obstruct drainage of the frontal sinus.

As dissection proceeds posteriorly, thick bone is encountered in the region of the orbital apex within 2 mm of the sphenoid face. This bone corresponds to the anulus of Zinn, from which the extraocular muscles originate and through which the optic nerve passes; this represents the posterior limit of a standard decompression. For patients with optic neuropathy, experienced surgeons may consider continuing the decompression posteriorly into the sphenoid sinus. The benefits of incorporating an optic nerve decompression into standard orbital decompression are unclear and may lead to inadvertent injury to the nerve. Anteriorly, fragments of bone are removed where the lamina papyracea joins the lacrimal bone. The thick white fascia of the lacrimal sac may be uncovered, but should not be opened. Thick bone anterior to the maxillary line covers much of the lacrimal sac and should not be removed.

Removal of the orbital floor may be the most technically challenging portion of the procedure. Only the portion of the floor medial to the infraorbital nerve is removed. A spoon curet is used to engage the orbital floor at its medial extent and down-fracture the bone (Fig. 3). The bone of the orbital floor

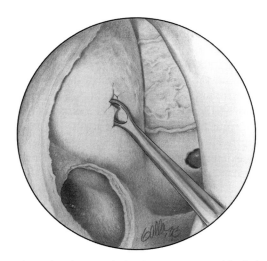

Fig. 2. A spoon curet is used to fracture the lamina papyracea and begin bony decompression.

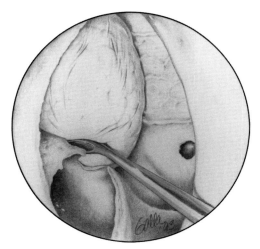

Fig. 3. A spoon curet is used to down-fracture the orbital floor. Inferior decompression continues laterally to the infraorbital canal.

is thicker than that of the medial orbital wall, and significant force is required for this maneuver. The spoon curet may not be sturdy enough for this portion of the procedure, and a more robust mastoid curet may be used. The bone may fracture in one large piece, typically with a natural cleavage plane at the canal of the infraorbital nerve. If it fractures into several small pieces, a 30° endoscope and curved instrumentation may facilitate bone removal, while preserving the infraorbital canal as the lateral limit of dissection.

When the lamina papyracea and medial orbital floor have been removed, the periorbita is fully exposed. A sickle knife may be used to open the periorbita (Fig. 4). Care must be taken to avoid "burying" the tip of the sickle knife and potentially injuring the underlying orbital contents, such as the medial rectus muscle. The use of a Steri-strip to cover all but the distal 2 mm of the knife may prevent deeper penetration. The periorbital incision should be initiated at the posterior limit of decompression (just anterior to the sphenoid face) and brought anteriorly so that prolapsing fat does not obscure visualization. Parallel incisions are performed along the ethmoid roof and orbital floor. To minimize the risk of postoperative diplopia, a sling of fascia overlying the medial rectus muscle may be preserved, while the remainder of the periorbita is removed using angled Blakesley forceps (Fig. 5) [5]. In patients with optic neuropathy, the fascial sling technique is not used to allow maximal decompression. A ball-tipped probe and sickle knife may be used to identify and incise remaining fibrous bands, which often course superficially between lobules of orbital fat. On completion of the procedure, a generous prolapse of fat into the opened ethmoid and maxillary cavities should be observed. The globe may be palpated to confirm a decrease in retropulsion.

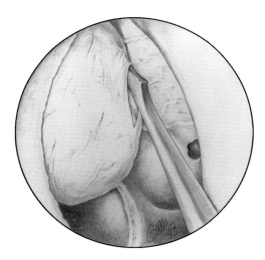

Fig. 4. A sickle knife is used to incise the periosteum. Care is taken to control the tip of the knife and prevent injury to the deeper orbital structures.

Depending on the clinical scenario and desired degree of decompression, a lateral decompression may be performed concurrently. When performed immediately after medial decompression, the orbital contents are retracted easily in a medial direction allowing for excellent exposure of the lateral bony wall. Concurrent excision of intraconal fat also may be performed if

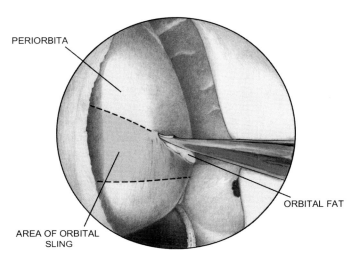

Fig. 5. A sling of periorbita overlying the medial rectus muscle may be preserved to minimize the risk of postoperative diplopia. This sling technique is not used in cases of optic neuropathy where decompression of the orbital apex is desired.

deemed necessary. Bilateral decompressions may be performed concurrently or in a staged procedure.

Nasal packing is avoided to ensure maximal decompression and avoid compression of exposed orbital contents. The patient is discharged the morning after surgery with a prescription for oral antibiotics and instructions to begin twice-daily nasal saline irrigations. At the first postoperative visit, 1 week after surgery, crusting is cleaned from the surgical site under endoscopic guidance.

For patients with severe comorbidities, with a strong preference for local anesthesia, or in whom surgery is being performed on an only seeing eye, decompression may be accomplished under local anesthesia with sedation [6]. This approach allows the surgeon to monitor the patient's vision throughout the procedure. Sedation may be achieved with an intravenous bolus of propofol (0.4–0.8 mg/kg) before injection of local anesthesia, followed by an infusion of 75 to 95 µg/kg during the procedure. Local anesthesia is administered initially with 4% cocaine pledgets followed by injection of lidocaine 1% with 1:100,000 epinephrine as described for patients undergoing general anesthesia. Patients often report discomfort during removal of the lamina papyracea. This sensation may be relieved by infiltration of a small amount of additional anesthetic solution into the periorbita.

Results

The goals of orbital decompression vary depending on the indication for the procedure. In patients with compressive optic neuropathy, restoration of visual deficits is the key outcome, whereas in patients with corneal exposure or severe proptosis, ocular recession may be the primary end point. The rate of improvement after endoscopic orbital decompression for Graves' orbitopathy ranges from 22% to 89% [1,7,8]. This wide variation in results reflects the diverse patient populations and definitions of improvement. Postoperative deterioration of visual acuity occurs in less than 5% of patients [2,7,8]. Ocular recession as a result of endoscopic decompression alone averages 3.5 mm (range 2–12 mm). The addition of concurrent lateral decompression to the endoscopic procedure provides an additional 2 mm of globe recession [8].

Complications

Diplopia is a frequent complication of orbital decompression with 15% to 63% of postoperative patients reporting new-onset diplopia or worsening of preexisting symptoms [2,6,8–11]. This complication is believed to be a result of a change in the vector pull of the extraocular muscles. Decompressive surgery rarely alleviates preexisting diplopia. Patients who have diplopia after decompressive surgery frequently require strabismus surgery for correction. All patients should be informed of the possibility of postoperative double vision and the potential for further surgical intervention.

Several methods to decrease postoperative diplopia have been reported. Multiple authors have described the preservation of a strut of inferomedial bone between the decompressed floor and medial wall [7,12]. When this strut is maintained, however, it is technically difficult to remove any of the orbital floor through a purely endoscopic technique. The maintenance of a facial sling in the region of the medial rectus has been shown to decrease postoperative diplopia [5]. This technique provides similar support as the medial strut technique, but allows for endoscopic access to decompress the medial orbital floor. The concept of a balanced decompression (concurrent medial and lateral decompression) also has been suggested as a means to decrease postoperative diplopia [9,13,14]. When operating for compressive optic neuropathy, techniques designed to limit diplopia also may limit the extent of decompression, and postoperative diplopia often is accepted as a concession to improved visual acuity.

Postoperative bleeding after decompression is best approached through endoscopic identification and direct cauterization of the bleeding site. Nasal packing generally is not used to avoid pressure on the exposed orbital apex and optic nerve. Postoperative infection is minimized through the use of postoperative antibiotics with staphylococcal coverage. A large maxillary antrostomy and limited bone removal in the frontal recess region minimize the risk of developing postoperative sinusitis. Epiphora may develop if the maxillary antrostomy is extended too far anteriorly with transaction of the nasolacrimal duct. This complication may be treated readily with an endoscopic dacryocystorhinostomy. Leakage of cerebrospinal fluid (CSF) and blindness are rare complications that have been reported primarily after nonendoscopic decompression techniques.

Endoscopic optic nerve decompression

Historically, the most frequent indication for optic nerve decompression has been traumatic optic neuropathy. More recent studies have questioned the role for decompression in these patients [15,16]. Currently, the most favorable indications for optic nerve decompression seem to be direct compression from fibro-osseous lesions or tumors [17–21]. Traditional surgical approaches for optic nerve decompression include transorbital, extranasal transethmoidal, transantral, intranasal microscopic, and craniotomy approaches. Endonasal endoscopic decompression of the optic nerve offers many advantages over these approaches, including excellent visualization, preservation of olfaction, rapid recovery time, lack of external scars, and less operative stress in patients who may have multisystem trauma.

Surgical anatomy

The optic nerve may be divided into three segments: intraorbital, intracanalicular, and intracranial. The goal of optic nerve decompression is to relieve compressive forces within the intracanalicular portion of the nerve. The canal of the optic nerve is formed by the two struts of the lesser wing of the sphenoid and carries the optic nerve and the ophthalmic artery. Within the optic canal, the nerve is encased by three meningeal layers: pia, arachnoid, and dura mater. At the orbital apex is the fibrous anulus of Zinn. This thick, fibrous layer is the least expandable portion of the fibrous tissue around the optic nerve and has been suggested to be the most susceptible site for pathologic compression [22,23].

Technique

Patients are prepared for surgery in a similar manner to patients undergoing orbital decompression. A standard sphenoethmoidectomy is performed. The sphenoid face is opened widely, and the bulge of the optic nerve canal is identified along the lateral wall of the sphenoid sinus, superior to the carotid artery. In some patients, the optic canal may be identified initially in a posterior ethmoid or Onodi cell, which can be identified on preoperative CT scan [24]. Identification and opening of the Onodi cell is important to provide adequate surgical exposure and allow full access to the optic canal.

After complete sphenoethmoidectomy, a spoon curet is used to fracture the lamina papyracea approximately 1 cm anterior to the optic canal. The lamina is removed carefully in a posterior direction to expose the annulus of Zinn. Care must be taken to avoid penetration of the periorbita because subsequent herniation of orbital fat obscures the surgical field. As the optic canal is approached, the thin lamina is replaced with the thick bone of the lesser wing of the sphenoid. This bone must be thinned before removal. A long-handled drill with a diamond burr is used methodically to thin the medial bone of the optic canal. While drilling, care must be taken to prevent contact of the drill bit with the prominence of the carotid artery, which is located just inferior and posterior to the optic nerve. After the bone is appropriately thinned, a microcuret is used to fracture the thinned bone in a medial direction, away from the optic nerve. Controversy exists as to the extent of bone that must be removed to achieve satisfactory decompression. For cases of traumatic optic neuropathy and dysthyroid orbitopathy, removal of bone for a distance of 1 cm posterior to the face of the sphenoid sinus is usually sufficient.

The authors generally do not recommend incision of the optic sheath in addition to bony decompression. Not only does this maneuver risk damage to the underlying nerve fibers and the ophthalmic artery, but also the risk of CSF leak and meningitis is increased. In select cases in which compression within the sheath is strongly suggested, such as with intrasheath hematoma or significant papilledema, opening of the optic nerve sheath may play a role.

When opening the optic nerve sheath, a sickle knife is used to incise the sheath just anterior to the anulus of Zinn. The sheath should be entered in its superomedial quadrant to minimize risk to the ophthalmic artery. The incision in the sheath may be continued posteriorly with the sickle knife or with microscissors. Some authors suggest the application of fibrin glue to the incision site after decompression to minimize the risk of CSF leak [17].

Results

The efficacy of optic nerve decompression in traumatic optic neuropathy is unclear. With the significant rate of visual improvement with observation alone, well-designed prospective studies are necessary to comment definitively on the efficacy of this procedure. Despite significant efforts, such studies have not been performed, largely owing to the rarity of this condition. This lack of randomized prospective data is unlikely to change, and clinicians are left to draw conclusions from uncontrolled and often contradictory retrospective reports.

Complications

The risk of CSF leak, meningitis, and visual loss with optic nerve decompression seems to be significantly higher than with standard endoscopic sinus surgery or orbital decompression. Although several studies report no complications in study sizes ranging from 20 to 45 patients, several more recent studies have reported CSF leaks, some with associated meningitis and visual decompensation [15,25].

Summary

Endoscopic orbital and optic nerve decompression are advanced techniques that should be performed only by surgeons experienced in endoscopic nasal surgery. The use of a transnasal endoscopic approach for these procedures allows for excellent visualization of the critical anatomy and avoidance of external scars. Although the benefits of orbital decompression have been well established, the role of optic nerve decompression remains controversial.

References

[1] Kennedy DW, Goodstein ML, Miller NR, Zinreich SJ. Endoscopic transnasal orbital decompression. Arch Otolaryngol Head Neck Surg 1990;116:275–82.
[2] Michel O, Bresgen K, Russmann W, et al. [Endoscopically-controlled endonasal orbital decompression in malignant exophthalmos]. Laryngorhinootologie 1991;70:656–62.
[3] Gorman CA, Garrity JA, Fatourechi V, et al. A prospective, randomized, double-blind, placebo-controlled study of orbital radiotherapy for Graves' ophthalmopathy. Ophthalmology 2001;108:1523–34.
[4] Mourits MP, van Kempen-Harteveld ML, Garcia MB, et al. Radiotherapy for Graves' orbitopathy: randomised placebo-controlled study. Lancet 2000;355:1505–9.

[5] Metson R, Samaha M. Reduction of diplopia following endoscopic orbital decompression: the orbital sling technique. Laryngoscope 2002;112:1753–7.
[6] Metson R, Shore JW, Gliklich RE, Dallow RL. Endoscopic orbital decompression under local anesthesia. Otolaryngol Head Neck Surg 1995;113:661–7.
[7] Schaefer SD, Soliemanzadeh P, Della Rocca DA, et al. Endoscopic and transconjunctival orbital decompression for thyroid-related orbital apex compression. Laryngoscope 2003; 113:508–13.
[8] Metson R, Dallow RL, Shore JW. Endoscopic orbital decompression. Laryngoscope 1994; 104:950–7.
[9] Shepard KG, Levin PS, Terris DJ. Balanced orbital decompression for Graves' ophthalmopathy. Laryngoscope 1998;108:1648–53.
[10] Wright ED, Davidson J, Codere F, Desrosiers M. Endoscopic orbital decompression with preservation of an inferomedial bony strut: minimization of postoperative diplopia. J Otolaryngol 1999;28:252–6.
[11] Eloy P, Trussart C, Jouzdani E, et al. Transnasal endoscopic orbital decompression and Graves' ophthalmopathy. Acta Otorhinolaryngol Belg 2000;54:165–74.
[12] Goldberg RA, Shorr N, Cohen MS. The medical orbital strut in the prevention of postdecompression dystopia in dysthyroid ophthalmopathy. Ophthal Plast Reconstr Surg 1992; 8:32–4.
[13] Unal M, Leri F, Konuk O, Hasanreisoglu B. Balanced orbital decompression combined with fat removal in Graves ophthalmopathy: do we really need to remove the third wall? Ophthal Plast Reconstr Surg 2003;19:112–8.
[14] Graham SM, Brown CL, Carter KD, et al. Medial and lateral orbital wall surgery for balanced decompression in thyroid eye disease. Laryngoscope 2003;113:1206–9.
[15] Levin LA, Beck RW, Joseph MP, et al. The treatment of traumatic optic neuropathy: the International Optic Nerve Trauma Study. Ophthalmology 1999;106:1268–77.
[16] Levin LA, Baker RS. Management of traumatic optic neuropathy. J Neuroophthalmol 2003; 23:72–5.
[17] Luxenberger W, Stammberger H, Jebeles JA, Walch C. Endoscopic optic nerve decompression: the Graz experience. Laryngoscope 1998;108:873–82.
[18] Sofferman RA, Harris P. Mosher Award thesis. The recovery potential of the optic nerve. Laryngoscope 1995;105:1–38.
[19] Plotnik JL, Kosmorsky GS. Operative complications of optic nerve sheath decompression. Ophthalmology 1993;100:683–90.
[20] Wax MB, Barrett DA, Hart WM Jr, Custer PL. Optic nerve sheath decompression for glaucomatous optic neuropathy with normal intraocular pressure. Arch Ophthalmol 1993;111: 1219–28.
[21] Sofferman RA. Transanasal approach to optic nerve decompression. Oper Tech Otolaryngol Head Neck Surg 1991;2:150–6.
[22] Anand VS, Al-Mefty C. Optic nerve decompression via transethmoid and supraorbital approaches. Oper Tech Otolaryngol Head Neck Surg 1991;2:157–66.
[23] Lang J. Anatomy of optic nerve decompression and anatomy of the orbit and adjacent skull base in surgical anatomy of the skull base. Berlin: Springer; 1989. p. 19.
[24] Allmond L, Murr AH. Clinical problem solving: radiology. Radiology quiz case 1: opacified Onodi cell. Arch Otolaryngol Head Neck Surg 2002;128:596, 598–9.
[25] Thakar A, Mahapatra AK, Tandon DA. Delayed optic nerve decompression for indirect optic nerve injury. Laryngoscope 2003;113:112–9.

ELSEVIER
SAUNDERS

Otolaryngol Clin N Am
39 (2006) 563–583

OTOLARYNGOLOGIC
CLINICS
OF NORTH AMERICA

Endoscopic Pituitary Surgery

Dharambir S. Sethi, MD, FRCSEd*,
Jern-Lin Leong, FRCS (Glasg)

*Department of Otolaryngology, Singapore General Hospital,
Outram Road, Singapore 169609, Republic of Singapore*

The sublabial transsphenoidal route for surgery on sellar lesions was described as early as 1907 [1]. However, this approach fell into disfavor because of the high incidence of complications and deep narrow exposure with poor illumination.

The introduction of the operating microscope a few decades later provided improved illumination and magnification. In 1958, Guiot [2] introduced radiofluoroscopy to visualize the depth and position of the surgical instruments intraoperatively. The use of the operating microscope combined with radiofluoroscopy was subsequently described [3]. The sublabial transseptal transsphenoidal approach using the operating microscope became the standard approach for pituitary tumors.

The operating microscope provided binocular three-dimensional vision and allowed use of both hands during surgery. In the 1980s endoscopes were introduced for nasal and paranasal sinus surgery [4,5]. The optical illumination and visualization provided by the endoscopes were unparalleled. By the late 1980s endoscope-assisted sinus surgery had gained popularity. Endoscopes not only revolutionized the way sinonasal pathology is treated but also helped establish a better understanding of the anatomy of the paranasal sinuses. Another major contribution was the introduction of CT for studying the paranasal sinuses, which provided radiologic details previously unavailable [6]. Called the *neglected sinus* for most of the past century, the sphenoid sinus in the last 2 decades generated a lot of interest and soon became the gateway for endoscope-assisted pituitary surgery.

In 1992, Jankowski and colleagues [7] first described the successful endonasal endoscopic resection of pituitary adenomas in three patients.

---

* Corresponding author.
E-mail address: goldss@sgh.com.sg (D.S. Sethi).

In 1994, we started performing endoscope-assisted pituitary surgery at our institution. Our earlier reports described the endoscopic transseptal transsphenoidal approach [8,9]. This approach was used in more than 300 patients who had pituitary tumors. Although the results were encouraging, this approach was limited because we had to work through a narrow tunnel created by elevating bilateral mucoperichondrial flaps on the nasal septum, removing the posterior nasal septum and sphenoid rostrum. Although visualization was not compromised because endoscopes provide excellent illumination, angled views, and a panoramic perspective of the sphenoid sinus, sella turcica, and related structures, instrumentation was often difficult, particularly when situations required two surgeons to work together while removing the tumor.

We modified our approach to overcome these limitations, and this article describes our current approach. This direct endoscopic endonasal approach has been used successfully in the past 6 years on more than 200 patients who had pituitary tumors.

Twelve years ago, our center was one of the few that started using endoscopes for pituitary surgery. Interestingly and encouragingly, the technique has gained wide acceptance [10–12].

Surgical anatomy

A good understanding of the anatomy of the sphenoid sinus and the sellar and parasellar region is essential before undertaking this surgery. Before performing this surgery, we studied the anatomy of this region in 30 cadavers [13]. A brief account of the surgical anatomy is presented.

Based on the extent of its pneumatization, the sphenoid sinus has been classified into three types; conchal, presellar, and sellar. In the conchal type the area below the sella is a solid block of bone without an air cavity. In the presellar type the air cavity does not penetrate beyond the coronal plane defined by the anterior sellar wall. In the sellar type the air cavity extends into the body of the sphenoid below the sella and may extend as far posterior as the clivus. The sellar type occurs in 86% of individuals [14]. The conchal type is very common in children younger than 12 years because pneumatization begins within the sphenoid sinus after the age of 12 years [15].

The ostium of the sphenoid sinus is located in the sphenoethmoid recess and varies in size from 1 to 4 mm. In most cases it can be identified medial to the superior turbinate about 1.5 cm superior to the posterior choana. Superiorly, it lies a few millimeters from the cribriform plate [14].

The pattern of the intersinus septa in the sphenoid sinus is variable. A single midline septum may extend posterior onto the anterior wall of the sella. More than one incomplete septae (accessory septae) are often present. The intersinus septae or the accessory septae may terminate onto the carotid canal in 40% of individuals and onto the optic nerves in 4%.

The lateral wall of the sphenoid sinus is related to the cavernous sinus that extends from the orbital apex to the posterior clinoid process. The cavernous sinus is formed by the splitting of the dura. The cavernous sinus contains delicate venous channels; the cavernous part of the internal carotid artery; the third, fourth, and the sixth cranial nerves; and fibro-fatty tissue. The internal carotid artery is the most medial structure within the cavernous sinus and forms a discernible prominence on the posterolateral aspect of the lateral wall of the sphenoid sinus. This prominence is well identified when the sphenoid sinus is well pneumatized. On the anterosuperior aspect of the lateral wall of the sphenoid sinus is another bulge formed by the optic nerve as it traverses the optic canal from the optic chiasma to the orbital apex. The prominence of the internal carotid artery is separated from the bulge of the optic nerve by a dimple on the lateral wall of the sphenoid sinus called the *opticocarotid recess*. The optic nerve and cavernous carotid artery are separated from the sphenoid sinus by a very thin bone. Dehiscence of these structures has been noted to be 4% and 8%, respectively [16]. In a well-pneumatized sphenoid sinus, the pterygoid canal and a segment of the maxillary division of the trigeminal nerve may be identified in the lateral recess of the sphenoid sinus.

The roof of the sphenoid (also known as the *planum sphenoidale*) anteriorly is in continuum with the roof of the ethmoid sinus. At the junction of the planum sphenoidale and the posterior wall of the sphenoid, the sphenoid bone is thickened to form the tuberculum sella. Inferior to the tuberculum sella, on the posterior wall, is the sella turcica, which forms a midline bulge. The sellar wall is approximately 0.5 to 1 mm thick [16]. It may be thinner inferiorly on the anterior sellar wall. Often the dura may be visible through this thin bone, imparting a bluish hue to the anterior sellar wall that aids in its recognition. Removal of the anterior sellar inferiorly provides access to the sella turcica.

The main portion of the pituitary gland lies in the sella turcica and is connected to the brain by the infundibulum. The diaphragma sella forms a dural roof for the greater part of the pituitary gland and is pierced by the infundibulum. In front of the infundibulum, the upper aspect of the gland is related directly to arachnoid and pia and the subarachnoid space here extends below the diaphragm, which is an important anatomic consideration while opening the anterior wall of the sella for access to the pituitary tumor. The pituitary gland is related above to the optic chiasma and below to an intercavernous sinus. Inadvertent intraoperative trauma to the intercavernous sinus may cause cumbersome bleeding. The structure is best avoided when extending the sellar opening inferiorly.

Preoperative and perioperative evaluation

Patients who have pituitary tumors usually present with endocrinologic and visual symptoms. Therefore, our referral base comes mainly from the departments of endocrinology and ophthalmology. All patients are discussed preoperatively at the "pituitary board" that comprises specialists from these disciplines. Complex cases, postoperative results, and complications are audited during these meetings. All patients undergo endocrine evaluation and visual field assessment pre- and postoperatively.

Indications for surgery include secretory and nonsecretory pituitary tumors. Nonsecretory tumors may grow large before becoming symptomatic. They often present with visual symptoms resulting from compression of the optic chiasma and oculomotor dysfunction, usually caused by involvement of the cavernous sinus. Most prolactin-producing pituitary tumors respond to bromocriptine. Surgery is reserved for patients who do not experience response, who are unable to tolerate medical treatment, and who have cystic tumors. Tumors secreting growth and adrenocorticotrophic hormones are indications for surgery to achieve endocrinologic cure.

A radiologic evaluation, including CT scans and MRI, is important for planning the transsphenoidal route. The extent of sphenoid pneumatization, sphenoid dominance, and internal sinus septae and their termination on the optic nerve or the internal carotid artery are important anatomic considerations. A presellar type of sphenoid sinus may be a relative contraindication to endoscopic transsphenoidal approach.

Preoperative endoscopic examination and treatment of nasal and paranasal sinus infections until the patient experiences a complete return to normal health is essential. Perioperative prophylactic antibiotics are routinely used. Some diseases can mimic pituitary adenomas. When an aneurysm is suspected, angiography should be considered. The differential diagnosis of meningioma, craniopharyngioma, and empty sella syndrome should also be considered.

Before the patient undergoes surgery, the surgical procedure, options and alternatives, and predicted outcome are discussed in detail and informed consent is obtained.

The authors' endocrinologist assists with the care of the patient during the entire perioperative period. Approximately 1 week after operation, baseline pituitary hormone function is again studied and appropriate replacement initiated.

Surgical setup

Fig. 1 shows the operative setup. The surgery is performed with the assistance of a neurosurgeon. The ear, nose, and throat (ENT) surgeon stands on the right side of the operating table and the neurosurgeon on the left (Fig. 2). The video camera system is placed at the cephalic end of the table to allow both surgeons to view the video monitor. The anesthetist is at the caudal end of the table. The scrub nurse and the instrument trolley are at the left cephalic end. Imaging studies are displayed for intraoperative reference.

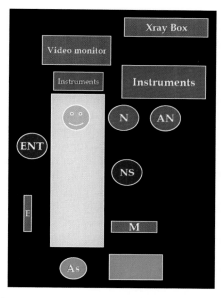

Fig. 1. The layout of the surgical setup for endoscopic pituitary surgery. ENT, ear, nose, and throat surgeon; NS, neurosurgeon; As, anesthesiologist; N, scrub nurse; AN, assistant nurse; E, Endoscrub [Medtronic Xomed, Jacksonville, Florida; M, microdebrider.

A three-chip video camera is attached to the eyepiece of the telescope and the entire procedure is monitored on a 14-inch high-resolution RGB video monitor. Video documentation of the surgical procedure is routinely performed on a digital video recorder. A powered sinus dissection device is used for the sphenoidotomy. We use the microdebrider developed by Medtronic. A 4-mm bit with a serrated outer shaft is used for the dissection.

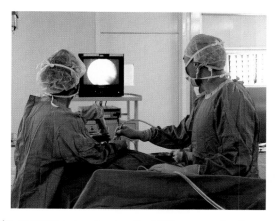

Fig. 2. View of the operating room showing the ENT surgeon standing on the right and the neurosurgeon on the left. The video monitor is at the cephalic end of the patient.

Surgical technique

Nasal preparation for surgery is similar to routine endoscopic sinus surgery. The nasal cavity is decongested by placing two neuropatties soaked in 4% cocaine in each side about 20 minutes before induction.

The patient is positioned supine on the operating table with the head elevated to 30°. The surgery is always performed under general anesthesia. Oral endotracheal intubation is used and a pharyngeal pack placed in the pharynx. Foley urinary catheter is routinely inserted to monitor urinary output intra- and postoperatively. Antiseptic solution (such as povidone) is applied to the nose and mouth, and the area draped with sterile towels and Steri-Drape (3M, ST. Paul, Minnesota). The lower abdomen is prepared and draped to obtain adipose tissue if necessary. Prophylactic antibiotic (cefazolin) is administered intraoperatively during induction.

The neuropatties that had been placed in the nasal cavity earlier are removed and discarded. The nasal cavity is once again decongested with topical application of cocaine. Sterile neuropatties soaked in 4% cocaine are endoscopically placed in the sphenoethmoid recess bilaterally. After allowing about 10 minutes for decongestion, the neuropatties are then removed and the sphenoethmoid recess is infiltrated bilaterally with 1% lidocaine with 1:80,000 epinephrine. A 21-gauge spinal needle is used for infiltration of the anterior wall of the sphenoid, sphenopalatine foramen, and posterior part of the nasal septum (Fig. 3).

The endoscope is held in the ENT surgeon's nondominant hand (left in our case) and the instruments in the dominant hand (right in our case). The neurosurgeon, standing on the left, holds suction and another instrument when necessary, particularly during tumor removal.

After the nose has been adequately decongested, an endoscopic examination is performed using a 0° or 30° endoscope. The sphenoid ostium is

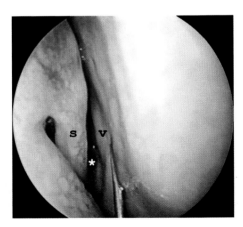

Fig. 3. Infiltration of the sphenoethmoid recess. The white asterisk indicates the sphenoid ostium. s, superior turbinate; v, vomer.

bilaterally identified in the sphenoethmoid recess (Fig. 4). Surgery is started on the side of the sphenoid ostium that is better visualized. Most of the time we start on the right side. The microdebrider with a 4-mm bit with a serrated outer shaft is used to debride the mucosa in the sphenoethmoid recess around the sphenoid ostium, taking care not to traumatize the mucosa on the superior turbinates. The serrated blade of the microdebrider is directed medially and the outer sheath laterally, protecting the mucosa of the superior turbinate. The sphenoid ostium is widened inferiorly and medially down to the floor of the sphenoid sinus. If the septal branch of the sphenopalatine artery is encountered it is cauterized with bipolar diathermy. If the bone of the sphenoid rostrum is thick, a 2-mm up- or down-biting Kerrison rongeurs may be used to extend the sphenoidotomy. Mucosa is débrided from the posterior part of the vomer and the sphenoid rostrum. The sphenoidotomy is extended to the contralateral side by dislocating the attachment of the vomer from the sphenoid rostrum. This maneuver is performed with a Freer elevator. The sphenoid ostium on the contralateral side is identified and the sphenoidotomy extended to contralateral superior turbinate by removing the sphenoid rostrum. A wide sphenoidotomy is created that extends superiorly to the roof of the sphenoid, inferiorly to the floor of the sphenoid sinus, and laterally to the superior turbinate on both sides. Approximately 1 cm of the posterior part of the vomer is removed with a reverse cutting forceps to facilitate unimpeded introduction of instruments from both nostrils (Fig. 5). The access to the sphenoid sinus is complete.

From this point, the ENT and neurosurgeon work as a team. The neurosurgeon introduces the suction through the left nostril to ensure an operating field that is not flooded with blood and the ENT surgeon controls the endoscope and other instruments. The sphenoid sinus is examined with

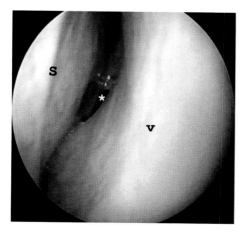

Fig. 4. Intraoperative endoscopic view of the sphenoid ostium (*asterisk*) (0° 4-mm endoscope). S, superior turbinate; v, vomer.

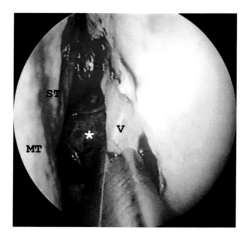

Fig. 5. The posterior part of the vomer (v) being removed. White asterisk indicates the location of the anterior wall of the sella. ST, superior turbinate; MT, middle turbinate.

0°, 30°, and 70° endoscopes and important anatomic landmarks within the sphenoid sinus are noted. Of particular importance are the structures on the lateral wall. The bulges of the cavernous carotid arteries and the optic nerves can be well identified when the sphenoid sinus is well pneumatized. On the posterior wall the tuberculum sella, the anterior wall of the sella and the clivus are identified. The location of the intersinus septae, if any, is noted. If these septae must be removed, extreme caution must be exercised because these often terminate on the carotid or optic canal. Through-cutting instruments are safer to use for removing these septae (Fig. 6). Injudicious avulsion of the septae with non–through-cutting instruments may cause

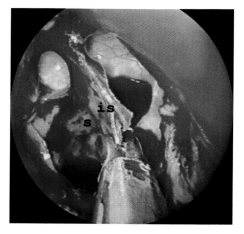

Fig. 6. The intersinus septum (is) being removed with a through-cutting straight Blakesley forceps. s, sella.

fracture of the thin bone overlying the cavernous sinus or optic nerve, resulting in hematoma, intractable bleeding, or even blindness. Caution is also advised to not strip the sphenoid mucosa because this may result in considerable bleeding. Once a panoramic view of the entire sphenoid sinus and surgical landmarks is obtained, the access to the sella turcica is complete.

A ball probe is used to gently assess the thickness of the anterior wall of the sella and the anterior sellar wall is fractured at its thinnest point. A plane is developed between the tumor capsule and the bony anterior sellar wall with a right-angle hook. A 1-mm Kerrison punch is used to delicately remove the bone of the anterior wall of the sella, exposing the dura or the tumor capsule (Fig. 7). The extent of the dura exposure is determined by the size of the tumor. Bipolar diathermy is used for hemostasis over the dura before incising it. A cruciate incision is often made. Care is taken not to extend the vertical segment of the incision too superiorly so as not to encounter the subarachnoid space. The intercavernous sinus should be avoided inferiorly and lateral extent is limited by the cavernous sinus on both sides. Generally, an opening large enough to admit a 4-mm endoscope pituitary forceps is sufficient.

The delivery of the tumor depends on the consistency of tumor contents. A cystic tumor will decompress rapidly. Large gelatinous or semisolid tumors are usually under pressure and decompress when the tumor capsule is incised (Fig. 8). Tumor tissue is taken for histologic examination. Once we have sufficient tumor tissue for a histologic examination, the tumor is removed using a combination of blunt ring curettes and pituitary forceps. The ENT and neurosurgeon work in tandem at this point. While one surgeon removes the tumor with a ring curette, the other provides continuous suction enabling rapid removal (Fig. 9).

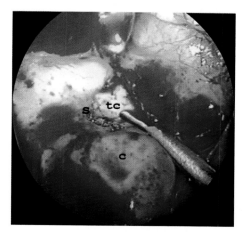

Fig. 7. The anterior wall of the sella turcica (s) being removed. tc, tumor capsule; c, clivus.

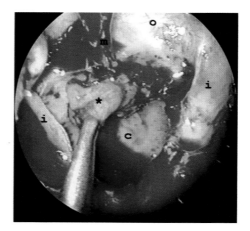

Fig. 8. Tumor (*black asterisk*) being removed with a blunt curette. i, accessory intersinus septae; m, midline intersinus septum (removed); o, left optic canal; c, clivus.

A systematic approach for removing the tumor is useful. We start to re- move the tumor from the floor, then from lateral extent, and finally from the suprasellar component (if any). Often the tumor decompresses rapidly in areas where it is cystic or gelatinous. The diaphragma may descend rapidly in this region, giving the impression that the tumor has been completely re- moved, whereas actually pockets of tumor where the tumor was more semi- solid or adherent to the diaphragma are left behind. We therefore attempt to control the descent of the diaphragma by systematic removal of the tumor. With the neurosurgeon standing on the left side, the trajectory of the instru- ments is favorable for removing the tumor from the right lateral aspect. For

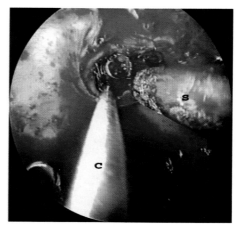

Fig. 9. Tumor is being removed with blunt curette and suction. At this point three instruments are in the surgical field: endoscope, straight suction (s), and blunt curette (c).

the same reason, the ENT surgeon removes the tumor from the left lateral aspect. The neurosurgeon removes tumor from 6 o'clock to 9 o'clock, then the ENT surgeon removes the tumor from 3 o'clock to 6 o'clock, then the neurosurgeon works again from 9 o'clock to 12 o'clock and the ENT surgeon from 12 o'clock to 3 o'clock. The surgeon must be gentle while working on the lateral aspect of the sella because the medial layer of the cavernous sinus can be extremely thin.

The suprasellar component, if any, is then removed. Blunt curettes are used because the arachnoid can be extremely thin and CSF leakage may result even with gentle manipulation. If the diaphragma descends unequally, a pocket of tumor may be left behind. In this situation one surgeon will gently retract the diaphragma away to enable visualization of the retained tumor. Once the tumor has been removed, a 4-mm angled endoscope at 30°, 45°, or 70° is used to examine the lateral and superior reaches of the sellar cavity for any remnant tumor, tumor capsule defect, CSF leakage, or dural defect (Fig. 10). A small tumor capsule defect without any CSF leakage is managed by lining the sella with a layer of Surgicel (Johnson & Johnson, New Brunswick, New Jersey) and fibrin glue. If a CSF leak is recognized intraoperatively, the defect is plugged with abdominal fat and fibrin glue. A subarachnoid catheter is placed postoperatively for 5 days to drain the CSF.

Once the surgery is concluded, hemostasis is ensured. Any minor oozing or bleeding from the septal branch of the sphenopalatine artery is controlled with bipolar application. To facilitate postoperative mucosal healing, care is taken to ensure that the bone of the sphenoid rostrum is adequately covered by mucosa. Eight-centimeter nasal Merocel sponges (Medtronic Xomed,

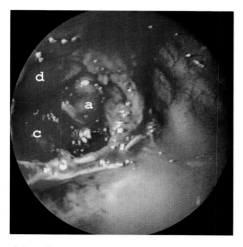

Fig. 10. Examination of the sellar cavity with 30° endoscope. a, cavernous carotid artery; c, clivus; d, diaphragma.

Jacksonville, Florida) are placed in the nasal cavity on either side, hydrated with saline to expand, and removed after 24 to 48 hours.

Postoperative care

The patient is monitored in the neurosurgical ICU for 24 hours after the surgery. The urinary catheter is removed after 24 hours if the patient does not develop diabetes insipidus. Nasal packing is removed on the first or second postoperative day and the patient is discharged on the second or third postoperative day. During the postoperative period the patient is monitored for any CSF leakage, symptoms and signs of meningitis, signs of hemorrhage, and any endocrinologic complications such as diabetes insipidus. Antibiotics and analgesics are routinely prescribed. The patient is examined after the packs are removed. Any blood clots in the nasal cavity are aspirated under endoscopic guidance.

The first office visit is scheduled for a week after the surgery. After application of topical 4% cocaine, blood clots are endoscopically removed from the nasal cavity and sphenoid sinus. The sella is carefully examined for any bleeding or CSF leakage. The patient is seen on a weekly basis by the ENT surgeon for the first 3 weeks and then every 3 weeks for the next two appointments. Healing usually takes about 3 to 6 weeks. Further appointments are scheduled as necessary. Postoperative follow-up is also provided by the endocrinologist, ophthalmologist, and neurosurgeon.

Results

We have performed approximately 200 endonasal endoscopic procedures for pituitary tumors using this technique and are in the process of collating our results. Figs. 11 through 17 show the pre- and postoperative MRI scans of two patients.

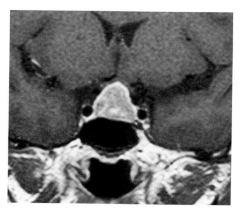

Fig. 11. Preoperative coronal MRI scans of a patient who has a nonsecretory pituitary tumor.

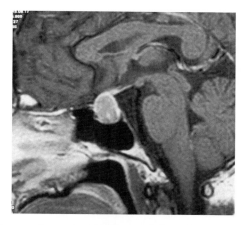

Fig. 12. Preoperative sagittal MRI scan of the patient shown in Fig. 11.

Complications

Endonasal endoscopic surgery for pituitary tumors is a minimally inva-sive, low morbidity procedure that is generally well tolerated by patients. However, complications may occur, including diabetes insipidus, CSF leak-age, bleeding, intrasellar hematoma, and even death. Our unpublished data of 158 patients who underwent surgery are shown in Table 1.

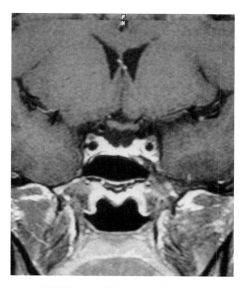

Fig. 13. Postoperative coronal MRI scan of the patient shown in Fig. 11 showing complete re-moval of the tumor.

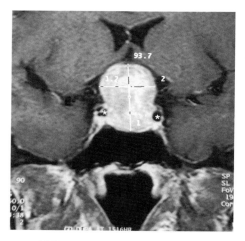

Fig. 14. Preoperative coronal MRI scan of a patient who presented with bitemporal hemianopia. MRI scan shows a pituitary tumor with a significant suprasellar extension. The white asterisk indicates the location of the cavernous carotid artery in the cavernous sinus.

Cerebrospinal fluid leakage

The most common intraoperative complication is CSF leakage. The usual cause of CSF rhinorrhea is trauma to the diaphragma resulting from instruments like curette, forceps or suction. The diaphragma may often be very thin and susceptible to trauma. Extreme caution must be exercised when

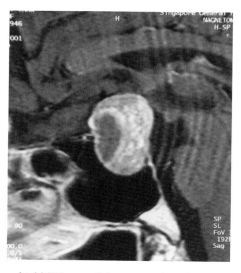

Fig. 15. Preoperative sagittal MRI scan of the same patient shown in Fig. 14. The tumor has a cystic and solid component.

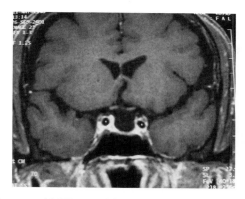

Fig. 16. Postoperative coronal MRI scan of the patient shown in Fig. 14 showing the complete removal of the tumor.

removing the tumor from this delicate structure. Surgeons must also remember that in front of the infundibulum, the upper aspect of the gland is related directly to arachnoid and pia, and the subarachnoid space here extends below the diaphragm and may be inadvertently breached while removing the tumor. Cappabianca and colleagues [17] report an intraoperative CSF leak in 90 of their 242 patients (37.1%) who underwent endonasal endoscopic pituitary surgery. In our series, only 14 (9%) patients of the 158 developed intraoperative CSF leak. When we identify a CSF leak intraoperatively, we try to identify the intrasellar defect. Extreme precaution is taken not to make it worse or larger and surgery is completed by working around it. At the conclusion of the surgery the defect is repaired with intrasellar placement of abdominal fat and fibrin glue. Lumbar drainage for 5 days is started postoperatively. In 5 of the 14 patients the CSF leak was caused by a minor "weeping" defect from the dura when the vertical component

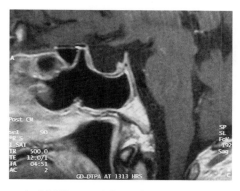

Fig. 17. Postoperative sagittal MRI scan of the patient shown in Fig. 14 showing complete removal of the tumor.

Table 1
Complications in the first 158 patients

	n	%
Diabetes insipidus	17	11
Hyponatremia	6	4
Intraoperative CSF leak	14	9
Postoperative CSF leak	0	0
Meningitis	0	0
Postoperative hemorrhage	5	3
Intrasellar hematoma	6	4
Deaths[a]	2	1

[a] One patient died of subarachnoid hemorrhage on the first postoperative day and another of myocardial infarction on the third postoperative day.

of the cruciate incision was extended superiorly. In these patients, we did not place any adipose tissue in the sellar cavity but repaired the weeping defect with a small amount of adipose tissue placed on the defect, fixing it with fibrin glue.

The incidence of CSF leakage after pituitary surgery ranges between 1.5% and 4.4% [18]. Cappabianca and colleagues [17] report an overall postoperative CSF leak rate of 2.06%. None of our patients developed a postoperative or postoperative persistence of CSF leak.

Meningitis

Meningitis is not a common complication after transsphenoidal surgery, but it can be fatal. The micro-organisms involved include *Staphylococcus aureus*, *Streptococcus pneumoniae*, and enteric organisms. Management should include broad-spectrum antibiotics and identification of the etiologic agent should be attempted through CSF cultures. None of our patients developed meningitis.

Diabetes insipidus

The incidence of diabetes insipidus as a complication of transsphenoidal surgery ranges from 0.4% to 17% [19]. It can be transient or permanent. Our incidence was 11% (see Table 1), and the condition was transient in all of our patients.

Once identified, diabetes insipidus is treated with intranasal administration of desmopressin acetate. Permanent diabetes insipidus probably represents pituitary stalk injury during surgery, and transient diabetes insipidus may be a result of excessive manipulation.

Bleeding

Intraoperative bleeding may result from inadequate nasal decongestion before surgery, inadvertent stripping of sphenoid mucosa, cavernous sinus trauma, intercavernous sinus injury, or trauma to the cavernous part of internal carotid artery.

Preoperative nasal preparation with cocaine and 1:80,000 epinephrine, the use of bipolar diathermy on the tumor capsule and the dura before incising it, and taking care to not strip the sphenoid mucosa are key factors in reducing intraoperative bleeding. Tumor tissue tends to bleed. Quick removal of tumor ensures early hemostasis. If bleeding continues from the sellar cavity, endoscopic examination with a 30° telescope is particularly useful in identifying the bleeding point or remnant tumor. The bleeding point can then be controlled with application of tamponade, bipolar diathermy, or a thin layer of Surgicel (Johnson & Johnson, New Brunswick, New Jersey).

Cavernous sinus bleeding should be suspected when venous bleeding fills the surgical field, and can be repaired with Surgicel and muscle and fibrin glue.

Perhaps the most feared complication is trauma to the cavernous carotid artery. Bleeding from the carotid artery should be suspected if the surgeon is working laterally.

Tamponade by promptly packing the nose and sinus cavity should be the initial measure taken to suppress this bleeding. Meanwhile, the patient's condition is assessed. If the blood loss has been heavy, the volume should be replaced. Blood pressure must be maintained to keep the brain perfused. Concurrently, arrangements should be made for angiography and balloon test occlusion of the internal carotid artery. If packing holds and the patient passes the occlusion test, the internal carotid artery may be permanently occluded with a balloon. However, if the patient fails the occlusion test, a bypass procedure is necessary before occluding the internal carotid artery. If the packing is unable to hold the bleeding, emergent measures such as occlusion of the internal carotid artery in the neck or a craniotomy may have to be undertaken.

None of our patients experienced trauma to the cavernous carotid artery.

Postoperative hemorrhage

Five of our cases developed postoperative hemorrhage. This complication was suspected when nasal packing could not hold the bleeding. Subsequent exploration under general anesthesia showed active bleeding from one of the branches of the sphenopalatine artery in two patients and generalized mucosal oozing from the mucosa over the remnant of the sphenoid rostrum in the other three. This hemorrhaging was controlled with application of bipolar cautery. Profuse bleeding that is difficult to control should alert one to the possibility of intracranial vascular trauma and warrant an angiogram.

Intrasellar hematoma

Transient or permanent worsening of vision may occur as a result of intrasellar hematoma or direct damage to optic nerve. Six of our patients developed intrasellar hematoma postoperatively. All had undergone surgery for large nonsecretory pituitary tumors with significant suprasellar extension. Intrasellar hematoma was suspected when patients complained of deteriorating vision approximately 18 hours after surgery. Emergent CT scan of the brain showed intrasellar hematoma in all cases. Immediate evacuation of the hematoma was performed and vision was restored to all patients. Some oozing from remnant tumor was noted during exploration. The remnant tumor was removed and bleeding from the tumor capsule was controlled with tamponade and lining the capsule with Surgicel. Excessive use of Surgicel to pack the sellar cavity is not recommended as this may aggravate intrasellar collection of the hematoma.

Death

Direct injury to the hypothalamus is the major cause of surgical death and occurs most often in patients who have large tumors characterized by significant intratumor bleeding.

Two of our patients died after surgery. One patient who had a very large nonsecretory tumor compressing on the ventricles experienced a subarachnoid hemorrhage approximately 24 hours after surgery. The other patient underwent successful surgery and was well until the third postoperative day when the patient experienced a massive myocardial infarction occurred and died of cardiogenic shock.

Discussion

We have discussed the advantages of the endoscopic transsphenoidal pituitary surgery in our earlier publications [8,9]. The excellent illumination, magnification. and visualization provided by the endoscopes offer a panoramic view of the surgical field during transsphenoidal surgery. The added advantage of angled vision assists in more complete tumor removal. Compared with the microscope, the smaller size of the endoscopic equipment enables it to quickly change the field of view between a close-up and a more panoramic perspective, allowing for constant monitoring of important surgical landmarks.

Critics of the endoscopic approach may highlight potential disadvantages of endoscopic surgery to include the lack of binocular viewing and subsequent lack of depth of field. However, depth perspective can be achieved through visual and tactile feedback, obtained while moving the telescope slightly in and out, together with palpation of structures with an instrument under endoscopic monitoring. This disadvantage is offset by the magnification and wider field of view available using an endoscope, because the field of view of the microscope is limited to the width of the defect in the face of the sphenoid.

Although our experience with the endoscopic transseptal transsphenoidal approach was very encouraging, instrumentation was often difficult, particularly when the situations required two surgeons to be working together while removing the tumor.

Additionally, an initial septoplasty requires a hemitransfixion incision, elevation of bilateral mucoperichondrial flaps, and removal of the posterior nasal septum. These maneuvers add to the morbidity of the surgical procedure. Infection, septal hematoma, perforation, and saddle deformity may result from a septoplasty, although these were not a major concern in our experience. The main difficulty the need to work through a narrow tunnel formed in the midline by elevation of the mucoperichondrial flaps. Although the passage was sufficient for introduction of the endoscope and instruments by the surgeon, it was inadequate when the same passage had to be shared by the surgeon and assistant.

The direct endonasal technique avoids a septoplasty and its inherent complications. No resection of the middle turbinate or superior turbinate for exposure is required. Occasionally if the middle or superior turbinates obscure the access to the sphenoid ostium in the sphenoethmoid recess, these may be gently retracted laterally for better exposure. We take the necessary precaution to avoid any mucosal trauma to the superior turbinates that form the lateral boundaries of the wide sphenoidotomy. The wide bilateral sphenoidotomies enable instrumentation from both sides. Continuous suction by the assistant enables a surgical field that is not flooded with blood. It also enables rapid tumor removal, reducing intraoperative bleeding and operative time. Retraction of the diaphragm sella by the assistant enables the surgeon to visualize the suprasellar extent of the tumor using angled endoscopes. This approach allows for greater teamwork between the ENT and neurosurgeon. We refer to this technique as the *four handed technique* because the ENT and neurosurgeon work in tandem with each other.

We do not use any self-retaining retractor or any endoscope holder. Use of a self-retaining retractor is unnecessary with this technique. Some surgeons use an endoscope holder and use two hands for instrumentation. We find one of the advantages of the endoscope to be the constant zooming in and out while removing the tumor, and fixing the endoscope limits that advantage.

One single factor that determines the outcome of this surgery is the consistency of the tumor. Although cystic and gelatinous tumors may be easily removed, the solid and fibrous ones may be challenging and complete removal may not be possible. Valsalva and irrigation may assist in tumor removal. Irrigation must be gentle and not forceful to avoid a CSF leak. One of the advantages of the four hand technique is when pockets of tumor are left behind because of rapid or uneven descent of the diaphragma. To enable visualization, one surgeon will control the endoscope and retract the diaphragma gently while the other surgeon uses a blunt curette and suction to look for residual tumor. At the end of the procedure the sella is repaired

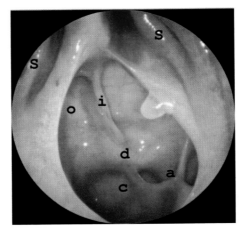

Fig. 18. Endoscopic (0°) postoperative view of the midline sphenoidotomy of patient in Fig. 12 taken 2 months after the procedure. The mucosa has healed completely. s, superior turbinate; d, sellar defect; a, bulge of the cavernous carotid artery; i, intersinus septum; c, clivus; o, right optic nerve.

if a CSF leak, prolapse of the suprasellar cistern, or bleeding from the cavernous or intercavernous sinus has occurred. The residual space in the sellar cavity is usually left free. Occasionally, if any minor oozing occurs from the sella, we place a thin layer of Surgicel over the area.

For invasive tumors with very large suprasellar extension a combined approach may be necessary. Complete removal may not be possible for tumors invading the cavernous sinus. Postoperative gamma knife ablation may be considered in such cases. No packing material is used for the sphenoid sinus.

Because the sphenoidotomy is left open, the postoperative mucosal healing of the sphenoid sinus is faster. A postoperative sphenoidotomy provides tumor surveillance and ready access if a reoperation is necessary (Fig. 18).

Summary

Endoscopic pituitary surgery has definite advantages over the traditional method using the operating microscope. Improved visualization, angled view, and a wider panoramic perspective of the important anatomic relationships of the sphenoid and the sella turcica are the obvious advantages. The direct endonasal transsphenoidal approach is the most minimally invasive. Its advantages include wider access, avoidance of a septoplasty, and the ability for two surgeons to work together, enabling better instrumentation and more complete and rapid removal of the tumor. We have been using this approach for the past 6 years and believe it will become the standard approach for endoscopic pituitary surgery.

References

[1] Schloffer H. Erfolgreiche operation eines hypophysen-tumors auf nasalem Wege. Wien Klin Wochenschr 1907;20:621–4.
[2] Guiot G. Transsphenoidal approach in surgical treatment of pituitary adenomas: general principles and indications in non-functioning adenomas. In: Kohler PO, Ross GT, editors. Diagnosis and treatment of pituitary tumors. Amsterdam: Series No. 303, Excerpta Medica, International Congress; 1973. p. 159–178.
[3] Hardy J. Microneurosurgery of the hypophysis: a subnasal transsphenoidal approach with television magnification and televised radiofluoroscopic control. In: Rand RW, editor. Microneurosurgery. St. Louis (MO): CV Mosby; 1969. p. 87–103.
[4] Kennedy DW. Functional endoscopic sinus surgery. Technique. Arch Otolaryngol 1985;111: 643–9.
[5] Stammberger H. Endoscopic endonasal surgery—concepts in treatment of recurring rhinosinusitis. Part II. Surgical technique. Otolaryngol Head Neck Surg 1986;94:147–56.
[6] Zinreich SJ, Kennedy DW, Rosenbaum AE, et al. Paranasal sinuses: CT imaging requirements for endoscopic surgery. Radiology 1987;163:769–75.
[7] Jankowski R, Auque J, Simon C, et al. Endoscopic pituitary tumor surgery. Laryngoscope 1992;102:198–202.
[8] Sethi DS, Pillay PK. Endoscopic management of lesions of the sella turcica. J Laryngol Otol 1995;109:956–62.
[9] Sethi DS, Pillay PK. Endoscopic pituitary surgery- a minimally invasive technique. Am J Rhinol 1996;10:141–7.
[10] Jho HD, Carrau RL. Endoscopic endonasal transsphenoidal surgery: experience with 50 patients. J Neurosurg 1997;87:44–51.
[11] Nasseri SS, Kasperbauer JL, Strome SE, et al. Endoscopic transnasal pituitary surgery: report on 180 cases. Am J Rhinol 2001;15:281–7.
[12] Cappabianca P, Alfieri A, de Divitiis E. Endoscopic endonasal transsphenoidal approach to the sella: towards functional endoscopic pituitary surgery (FEPS). Minim Invasive Neurosurg 1998;41:66–73.
[13] Sethi DS, Stanley RE. Endoscopic anatomy of the sphenoid sinus and sella turcica. J Laryngol Otol 1995;109:951–5.
[14] Lang J. Clinical anatomy of the nose, nasal cavity and paranasal sinuses. New York: Thieme; 1989.
[15] Mattox DE, Carson BS. Transpalatal trans-sphenoidal approach to sella in children. Skull Base Surg 1991;1:177–82.
[16] Fujii K, Chambers SM, Rhoton AL Jr. Neurovascular relationship of the sphenoid sinus— a microsurgical study. J Neurosurg 1979;50:31–9.
[17] Cappabianca P, Cavallo LM, Valente V, et al. Sellar repair with fibrin sealant and collagen fleece after endoscopic endonasal transsphenoidal surgery. Surg Neurol 2004;62:227–33.
[18] Welbourn RB. The evolution of trans-sphenoidal pituitary microsurgery. Surgery 1986;100: 1185–90.
[19] Laws ER Jr, Kern EB. Complications of trans-sphenoidal surgery. Clin Neurosurg 1976;23: 402–16.

ELSEVIER
SAUNDERS

Otolaryngol Clin N Am
39 (2006) 585–600

OTOLARYNGOLOGIC
CLINICS
OF NORTH AMERICA

Common Fibro-osseous Lesions of the Paranasal Sinuses

Robert Eller, MD[a], Michael Sillers, MD[b],*

[a]*American Institute for Voice and Ear Care and The Graduate Institute,
Philadelphia, PA, USA*
[b]*Alabama Nasal and Sinus Center, 7191 Cahaba Valley Road,
Birmingham, AL 35242, USA*

Within the broad spectrum of disease that can affect the paranasal sinuses is a class of benign bony abnormalities known collectively as fibro-osseous lesions. Fibrous dysplasia, ossifying fibroma, and osteoma are three distinct entities that lie along a continuum from the least to the most bony content. They have similar appearance and makeup; however, their clinical implications vary. This article focuses primarily on sinonasal osteomas, with less emphasis on fibrous dysplasia and ossifying fibroma.

History

Through the years, theories of the origin of bony lesions in the sinonasal and intracranial areas have evolved from that of vestigial horn-forming organs to petrified brain to bony tumors. Summers and colleagues [1] outline the history of sinonasal osteomas and credit Viega with the first documentation of a sinus osteoma, which Viega successfully removed in 1506. Later, Bartholinus and Du Verny documented other bony lesions in the frontal region, but conjectured that they were petrified brain. In 1733, Vallisnieri described a sinus osteoma that protruded into the brain, but asserted that it had a bony rather than a neural origin.

Epidemiology

Osteoma is the most common tumor of the paranasal sinuses. Its incidence is between 0.014% and 0.43% [2–8]. In 1999 Vowles and Bleach

* Corresponding author.
E-mail address: Michael.Sillers@ccc.uab.edu (M. Sillers).

0030-6665/06/$ - see front matter © 2006 Elsevier Inc. All rights reserved.
doi:10.1016/j.otc.2006.01.013

reviewed 3510 sinus radiographs and found an incidence of 0.43% [9]. Mahabir and colleagues [10] report the number seen on plain film as 0.25%. The true incidence may be higher, as the incidence on computed tomography of the head or sinuses has been reported as high as 3% [5,6].

There is a male predominance in most series [1, 5–8], with a male/female ratio that ranges from 1.5:1 to 3.1:1. Naraghi and colleagues [5] speculate that this is because men have larger sinuses and are more prone to facial trauma, one of the proposed etiologic theories. Age at diagnosis varies, but is predominantly the second and third decade, although patients can be diagnosed later in life [6]. There is no mention of racial predilection in the literature.

Etiology

There are three accepted theories of the etiology of paranasal sinus osteoma: developmental, traumatic, and infectious. No single theory adequately explains all osteomas.

Developmental theory

In the mid-nineteenth century, scientists formalized the concept that adult tissues contain embryonic remnants that generally lie dormant, but can activate to become a neoplasm [11]. The ethmoid bone is a result of endochondral bone formation, whereas the frontal bone is ossified by the membranous pathway. In the developmental theory, the apposition of membranous and endochondral tissues traps some of these embryonic cells, eventually leading to unchecked osseous proliferation [4]. This could explain lesions that develop near the frontoethmoidal suture lines, but does not account for osteomas that arise elsewhere. Naraghi and Kashfi [5] suggest the tumors could arise from rests of cartilage or osseous stem cells present in bone other than at suture lines, but little in the known histopathology points firmly in that direction.

Traumatic theory

The traumatic theory and the infectious theory are very similar. Both rely on an inflammatory process as the inciting force for bony tumor formation. There is moderate evidence for bony trauma as an inciting event. Moretti and colleagues [4] report that up to 20% of sinus osteomas follow some sort of trauma and present the case of an osteoma that developed in a maxillary sinus 9 years after a Caldwell-Luc procedure. Because the primary surgery was not performed by his group, it is unknown whether the lesion went undiagnosed during the original procedure. Sayan and colleagues [7] note that osteomas arising on the mandible have a predilection for places where muscles insert on the bone. In their view, minor trauma could incite an inflammatory process under the periosteum, which could persist as a result of the constant traction applied by the musculature. Several investigators feel that the increased incidence of trauma in males is responsible for the male predilection [5,7]. However, the traumatic theory fails to explain adequately lesions in older patients or those without a history of trauma.

Infectious theory

The infectious theory suggests that osteitis resulting from chronic infection is to blame. Data from Rawlins [12] from 1938 show a 28% incidence of infection coinciding with sinonasal osteoma. It is difficult to determine if the osteoma or the infection is the primary (or secondary) process. Indeed, tumor and infection frequently coexist at the time of diagnosis. In the senior author's clinical experience, an osteoma has never arisen in a patient with long-standing chronic rhinosinusitis. Furthermore, the type of bone in an osteoma (eburnated or spongy) differs significantly from the bony hyperplasia one would expect to characterize reactive osteitis.

Further research, possibly at the genetic level, is needed to be certain of what initiates osteoma formation.

Pathology

The surface of an osteoma is smooth and lobulated [2,6]. It may be sessile or pedunculated [2]. It is covered by the sinus mucosa. Histologically, there are three types of osteomas. The eburnated type, also known as the ivory or compact type, is very dense and lacks haversian canals [1,6]. It may arise from membranous elements. The mature type, or osteoma spongiosum, is composed of softer bone more similar to cancellous bone. It is thought to arise from cartilaginous elements [5]. Both are dense lamellar bone with little medullary component, containing fibro-fatty tissue in the interstices (Fig. 1) [6,13]. The mixed type of osteoma contains elements of both the eburnated and mature forms.

Natural history

If untreated, osteomas will continue to grow slowly during the life of the patient, but they are always benign. There are no reported cases of malignant degeneration or metastasis. Recurrence after complete resection is extremely rare; only a few cases have been reported [2,7].

Location

The vast majority (95%) of sinonasal osteomas are found in the frontoethmoidal region (see Refs. [1,2,4,6–8, 14]). More than 80% are in the frontal bone, arising from the floor of the frontal sinus [1,14]. Schick and colleagues [8] report a series of 23 frontal osteomas. Twelve originate

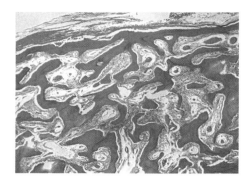

Fig. 1. Low-power photomicrograph of hematoxylin-eosin section of a paranasal sinus osteoma. (Original magnification – 10X).

from the posteroinferior wall of the frontal sinus, medial to the plane of the lamina papyracea. Eleven are lateral to this plane. This distinction is useful in determining the feasibility of endoscopic resection. Lateral tumors often require an external approach. The ethmoid sinuses account for 20% to 30% of sinus osteomas. The maxillary sinus is involved in less than 5% of cases, usually on the lateral wall of the sinus [4]. Sphenoid osteomas are distinctly rare [4,6]. Other reported sites of osteoma formation in the skull include the external auditory canal, the orbital bones, the temporal bone, the pterygoid plates, and the mandible, sphenoid and occipital bones [7].

Symptoms

Symptoms related directly to an osteoma generally arise from a "mass effect" as the lesion impinges on normal structures. As many as 60% of patients with frontal osteomas present with a chief complaint of headache (see Refs. [1,4,6,10,15,16]). The headache can be constant, episodic, mild, or severe. Other symptoms attributed to osteoma include diplopia, facial deformity, sinusitis symptoms, and dizziness. When an osteoma compromises ventilation and drainage from the associated sinus, acute or chronic rhinosinusitis may arise or a mucocele may develop over time [1,4,6]. Often, patients have been treated nonspecifically for "sinus" before subspecialty referral or radiographic evaluation.

Many patients diagnosed with an osteoma of the paranasal sinuses are asymptomatic. These lesions are discovered incidentally during radiographic evaluation for unrelated problems such as minor head trauma.

Radiology

Plain sinus radiographs are usually adequate for detecting osteomas, and between 0.25% and 1% of sinus films will demonstrate one [5,6,10].

However, computed tomography (CT) is more sensitive, with 3% of CT scans through the sinuses demonstrating an osteoma [5,6]. In either type of radiographic study, osteomas appear as very dense, homogeneous, well-circumscribed masses attached with an apparent range of broad to narrow pedicles to adjacent bone (Fig. 2). The surrounding bone is normal and does not have a lytic or moth-eaten appearance. Even for extensive osteomas, surrounding bone is thinned and moved by pressure rather than by direct invasion.

For patients with an osteoma where there is any question of extrasinus extension or intracranial involvement, MRI is recommended [1,14,17]. MRI is able to show dural involvement or transgression, and can distinguish mucoceles from neoplasms. Mucoceles vary in appearance with protein content, hydration, and viscosity. On T1 imaging with gadolinium, mucoceles usually have a thin peripheral linear enhancement with a low central signal [14]. Soft tissue neoplasms show more uniform enhancement, even with extensive central necrosis.

Complications from osteomas

Extrasinus complications can be divided into orbital and intracranial problems. Osteomas may expand slowly into the orbital vault, displacing the orbital contents. This may lead to diplopia, epiphora, facial distortion, and even blindness [1,2,6,8]. Removal of the osteoma usually restores normal vision. In rare instances of extreme expansion, the orbital vault requires reconstruction.

Intracranial complications occur when an osteoma penetrates the dura. These complications include mucoceles, meningitis, frontal abscess secondary to hematologic seeding across the bridging veins, cerebrospinal fluid (CSF) leak, or pneumatocele (see Refs. [1,3,8,10,13,17–20]). Overall,

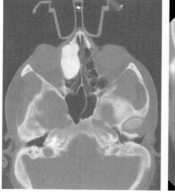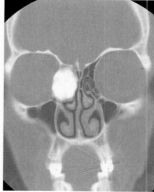

Fig. 2. Axial and coronal sinus CT images of an ethmoid osteoma.

mucoceles are present in 12% to 50% of osteoma cases [13]. However, there are less than 25 reported cases of intracranial mucoceles associated with osteomas [13,17]. It has been postulated that osteomas with mucoceles follow a more aggressive clinical course than those without mucoceles [17]. This may be because the mucocele expands at a faster rate than the typical osteoma, but Akay and colleagues [17] suggest that calcification of the mucocele can occur, leading to rapid expansion of the complex.

Meningitis and brain abscesses can result from direct intracranial osteoma or mucocele extension [1,17,18], but they can also be seeded from adjacent or nonadjacent sinuses [1,20]. Summers and colleagues [1] report a case of an osteoma contributing to maxillary sinusitis, which presumably seeded the veins in the "danger triangle" with subsequent cerebral abscess.

Two other possible problems are CSF leak and pneumatocele. Both of these can occur with a breach in the dura. They may occur independently or together. Seventy-five percent of pneumatoceles are secondary to surgery or trauma; only 13% are secondary to a tumor [3]. Johnson and Tan state that most of the 13% are accounted for by frontal and ethmoid osteomas. Air can become trapped in the cranial vault by two mechanisms. The first pathway is analogous to an inverted water bottle: air goes in when water goes out. Thus, after a rent is created in the dura, CSF flows out, creating a vacuum drawing air in. The second mechanism involves a valve and pressure. A rent in the dura is maintained in the closed position by the CSF pressure. When the extracranial pressure changes, such as during a sneeze, the flap is forced open and air is pushed into the intracranial space. Mahabir and colleagues [10] report a case where this was caused by air travel in a patient with an undiagnosed frontal osteoma, and Johnson and Tan [3] report a case of intraparenchymal tension pneumatocele with a frontal osteoma.

Management options

The primary dilemma in patients with osteoma is determining if surgical removal is indicated. Because the majority of osteomas are asymptomatic, observation with periodic re-evaluation is reasonable. Pain may or may not be related to an osteoma, especially if the locations of the pain and the osteoma are not congruent. Even when they do correspond, in some instances a thorough neurologic evaluation for pain may reveal another treatable cause, such as migraine. Since most osteomas are asymptomatic, many investigators advocate periodic imaging to follow growth and allow intervention before the development of complications [3]. Initially, a 3- to 6-month follow-up and an annual follow-up thereafter are recommended if no growth is detectable on CT and the patient remains asymptomatic. Patients should be educated about the potential for and nature of symptoms and should be instructed to seek evaluation if they change clinically. Acute complications, especially intracranial problems, must be managed by the professional most capable of normalizing the situation. The osteoma can be managed at the same time or after the patient is more stable.

Indications for operation

Most authors agree that small, asymptomatic lesions do not need surgery (Figs. 3 and 4) [1,3,4,6,8]. There is also agreement that symptomatic tumors should be removed. Rapid growth, infection, compression of vital structures, severe pain, and facial deformity are some of the possible symptomatic indications (Fig. 5) [4]. For example, if a patient complains of headache in the vicinity of an osteoma, and other pathology leading to headache has been ruled out, excision is indicated [8]. For larger asymptomatic lesions, or those that are certain to cause problems in the future, several investigators have developed guidelines. Summers and colleagues [1] and Johnson and Tan [3] recommend that if the tumor occupies more than 50% of the frontal sinus it should be removed, regardless of symptoms. Rappaport and Attia [21] suggest that posterior-based frontal lesions should be considered for early excision due to the increased likelihood of intracranial complications. Lesions in the frontal recess and any osteoma in the ethmoid cavity are also indications for removal [8].

Surgical techniques

Multiple surgical approaches have been described for removal of this neoplasm from the paranasal sinus. In general, approaches can be categorized as transnasal endoscopic, external, or combined. Regardless of the technique chosen, two primary tenets should be followed. First and foremost is the complete removal of the osteoma, which is the most important

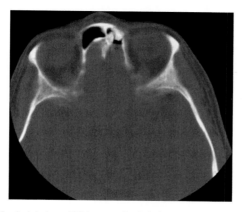

Fig. 3. Axial sinus CT image of a left frontal recess osteoma.

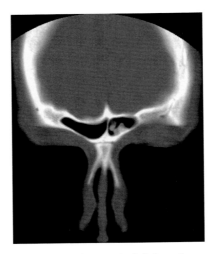

Fig. 4. Coronal sinus CT image of a left frontal recess osteoma.

step toward a cure. The second is minimizing trauma to the surrounding normal structures and to the sinonasal mucosa. This will result in more rapid healing and enable long-term endoscopic surveillance (Fig. 6).

The choice of a transnasal endoscopic, external, or combined approach is based on the size and location of the tumor. The authors agree that almost all ethmoid tumors are amenable to endoscopic removal (Figs. 7 and 8) [4,12]. To determine if the endoscopic approach is feasible for frontal sinus

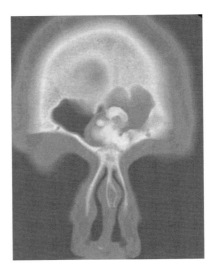

Fig. 5. Coronal sinus CT of a large frontal osteoma with obstructive sinusitis and mucocele formation.

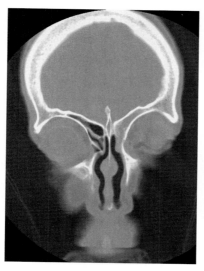

Fig. 6. Coronal sinus CT of a left frontal recess reactive bony hyperplasia after endoscopic drill out to remove osteoma with resultant frontal sinusitis.

lesions, Schick and colleagues [8] recommend that the anteroposterior diameter of the frontal sinus drainage pathway be measured to ensure that it is large enough for instrumentation. They recommend an appropriate ethmoidectomy and usually a Draf II or III procedure. Furthermore, they feel that lesions that are lateral to the sagittal plane of the lamina papyracea or that are anterior based should undergo an external osteoplastic procedure. Chen and colleagues [2] and Selva and colleagues [22] have similar recommendations and suggest that an endoscopic modified Lothrop procedure may be necessary to remove many frontal sinus lesions.

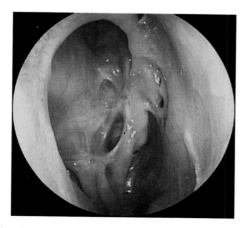

Fig. 7. Postoperative view of the ethmoid cavity after endoscopic removal of an osteoma.

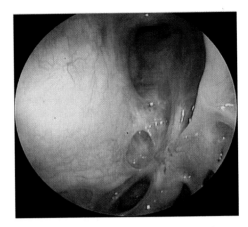

Fig. 8. Postoperative view of the frontal recess after endoscopic removal of an osteoma.

External approaches to the sinuses continue to evolve. Although the Lynch frontoethmoidectomy was once standard, it is used rarely now because of expected stenosis of the frontal recess. An osteoplastic flap is still very useful, and most agree that the coronal incision is cosmetically and neurologically superior to brow ("gull-wing") or midforehead approaches. Almost all investigators reporting on osteoma maintain the coronal osteoplastic flap as part of their surgical practice [2,4,6,8,22]. However, concomitant obliteration of the frontal sinus has become less common [8]. When intracranial complications occur, or when there is a large defect of the posterior frontal sinus wall, cranialization with obliteration of the frontal recess is recommended [3,13,17].

Some lesions lend themselves to combined endoscopic and external approaches. Frequently, endoscopic and osteoplastic flap procedures are combined to preserve frontal sinus health after tumor removal. A full osteoplastic flap procedure is not always necessary, and frontal trephines may be used for small symptomatic frontal sinus osteomas [23]. Chen and colleagues [2] and Selva and colleagues [22] report using orbital approaches to access difficult lesions, avoiding craniotomy in some cases.

The development of computer-aided surgery (CAS) in the last decade, combined with microdebrider technology, has enabled surgeons to remove extensive osteomas using transnasal endoscopic approaches. Previously, these tumors were simply too large to remove through the nasal cavity, and required an external approach. Now, by combining these two technologic advances, a large tumor can be reduced sufficiently before cleavage, while maintaining a safe relationship between the lesion and the skull base or lamina papyracea (Fig. 9). The position of the ethmoid roof and lamina papyracea are defined easily and accurately in several planes, allowing more safety in skull base and orbital dissection. The disadvantage, however, is that real-time confirmation of complete tumor removal is not possible from

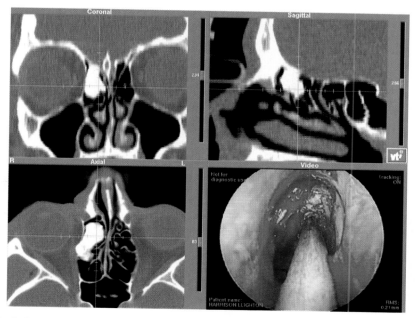

Fig. 9. Intraoperative screen capture obtained during surgical navigation performed for localization for endoscopic excision of a left ethmoid osteoma.

preoperative images alone. To account for this, Selva and colleagues [22] recommend also using stereotactic fluoroscopy during especially challenging cases where the real-time knowledge of spatial relationships is imperative.

Regardless of the approach used, violation of the skull base or bony orbit, while not common, should be anticipated. This is especially true when dividing the cleavage plane at the base of the bony tumor where it attaches to the lateral lamella of the cribriform plate or a significantly thinned ethmoid roof or lamina papyracea (Fig. 10). The resources and skill to reconstruct necessary defects should be in place prior to surgery. In patients with existing CSF leaks or apparent uncomplicated intracranial extension, lumbar drainage and neurosurgical support may be necessary.

Surgical complications

All of the known complications of sinus surgery are possible during resection of a paranasal sinus osteoma. Injury to the periorbita, optic nerve, cribriform plate, or other important structures is possible. However, in experienced hands, complications are rare. Schick and colleagues [8] report on the endoscopic removal of 23 tumors. They had three instances of minor injury to the periorbita without symptomatic complication, and three instances of injury to the dura. These were repaired endonasally at the time

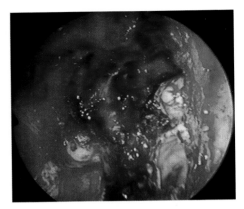

Fig. 10. Endoscopic view of orbital fat protrusion through an opening in the left medial orbital wall after orbital and optic nerve decompression for fibrous dysplasia.

of the initial surgery and there were no symptomatic complications noted. They also performed 11 osteoplastic flaps, and had four dural injuries and one injury to the periorbita, all without short- or long-term problems. Chen and colleagues [2] further report on the complications of osteoplastic flaps. In addition to CSF leak, frontal pain, and paresthesia/anesthesia, frontal bossing, and fracture or necrosis of the bone flap can occur.

With either endoscopic or external approaches, disruption of the sinus walls and violation of the mucosa can establish a reactive bony hyperplasia. This is commonly considered a reason for surgical failure in the frontal sinuses after functional endoscopic sinus surgery for chronic rhinosinusitis. Reactive bony hyperplasia should be distinguished from tumor recurrence and managed appropriately.

Postoperative course

Postoperative morbidity depends generally on the surgical approach used and whether or not the dura or periorbita were violated. When the dura and periorbita are uninjured, outpatient surgery with standard postoperative sinus care is adequate. For patients with significant orbital involvement, ophthalmologic evaluation is imperative both before and after surgery. If CSF rhinorrhea is encountered or repaired, lumbar drainage may be employed, but is often unnecessary. It is imperative that the patient be cared for by nursing staff familiar with lumbar drainage, as mismanagement can lead to significant morbidity and mortality.

Following discharge, the patient should return to the office on a weekly basis until all mucosal surfaces have healed. Monthly visits may be necessary to prevent and manage evolving stenosis. Once the area has stabilized, yearly visits with CT imaging for a total of three years are required to ensure continuing health and identify recurrent/persistent tumor.

Gardner's syndrome

There is one syndrome associated with sinus osteoma that should be considered when evaluating these patients. Gardner's syndrome, the triad of colorectal polyps, skeletal abnormalities, and supernumerary teeth, is also characterized by the presence of multiple osteomas. This disease is autosomal dominant and carries a 100% risk of malignant transformation of the colonic polyps by the age of 40. Thus, early diagnosis is important. Usually, patients become symptomatic in the second decade of life, with rectal bleeding, diarrhea, or abdominal pain [7]. Extracolonic manifestations can complicate treatment and increase morbidity [24]. It is important to investigate this possibility when taking the history of patients with osteomas and follow any leads with appropriate studies or referrals.

Fibrous dysplasia

Fibrous dysplasia (FD) is another slow-growing fibro-osseous lesion that can be located in the paranasal sinuses. Seventy-five percent of patients with FD are diagnosed before the age of 30 [19]. There are two forms: polyostotic (15%–30%), involving more than one bone, and monostotic (70%–85%), involving only one bone [25]. McCune-Albright syndrome (precocious puberty, fibrous dysplasia, café-au-lait spots) has the polyostotic form. Twenty-five percent of monostotic cases arise in the facial skeleton [16]. The maxilla and mandible are the most common sites in the head and neck, although it has been reported throughout the maxillofacial skeleton, including the sphenoid intersinus septum [12,25].

FD is generally assumed to "burn out" as the patient reaches skeletal maturity, although this is debated [16,19,25]. Monostotic FD in the long bones and mandible does not cross the joint line and is contained within the diseased bone. However, in maxillofacial skeleton, it can cross bony sutures and involve more than one facial bone. While disfiguring, FD has a low rate of malignant transformation [16,19,25]. However, transformation occurs in 0.5% of polyostotic forms and in 4% of lesions in patients with McCune-Albright syndrome [25].

In the paranasal sinuses, diagnosis can be accomplished via radiographic appearance, although some investigators recommend biopsy of FD lesions in the jaw [25]. In plain film and CT radiographs, FD lesions are characterized by hazy borders and a fairly homogeneous "ground glass" appearance representing the disorganized spicules of bone that characterize FD's histology (Fig. 11) [15,25]. As the lesion scleroses, "cotton wool" areas arise. On MRI, the T1 signal is intermediate and the T2 signal is hypointense [25].

Because FD has a tendency to stabilize over time and a low malignancy potential, most investigators recommend conservative management, operating only for symptomatic lesions or to recontour cosmetic deformity. In the paranasal sinuses, this is usually accomplished via an endoscopic technique,

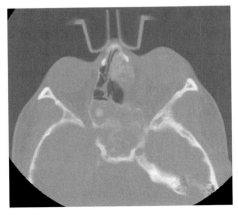

Fig. 11. Axial CT scan of fibrous dysplasia in the left ethmoid sinuses. Note the heterogeneous ground glass appearance.

and radical or complete resection is not necessary [12,19]. Patients should be followed up with periodic imaging to guide management of any regrowth that occurs.

Ossifying fibroma

Ossifying fibroma (OF) is the most concerning of the paranasal sinus's fibro-osseous lesions. Also known as cemento-ossifying fibroma, psammomatoid ossifying fibroma, and juvenile-aggressive ossifying fibroma, this lesion can be locally destructive. It involves the mandible in 75% of cases, but is considered more aggressive when found outside the mandible. Histologically, there are islands of osteoid rimmed by osteoblast-forming lamellar bone. The cellular fibrous stroma shows a parallel and whorl arrangement of collagen and fibroblasts [16]. Radiographically, it is a sharply circumscribed round or oval lesion with an eggshell rim and a central radiolucency. OF will absorb tooth roots, whereas FD usually encompasses the healthy roots [25]. Because of the aggressive and locally destructive nature of OF, complete removal is recommended.

Summary

Osteomas are the most common fibro-osseous lesions in the paranasal sinuses. They are infrequent, with an incidence of 0.43%, and are seen in up to 3% of sinus CT series. Histologically, they are made of dense lamellar bone without haversian canals, or otherwise mature bone. Thus, they appear radiographically as well-circumscribed dense masses attached to the originating bone by either a broad- or narrow-based pedicle. The three theories of pathogenesis are developmental, traumatic, and infectious. They may arise from residual cartilaginous rests or as a reaction to an inciting event. Most frequently, osteomas are asymptomatic and are discovered incidentally. When they do cause symptoms, headache is most frequent, followed by sinusitis, pain, and facial or cranial deformation. Complications arise when an osteoma has grown large enough to impinge on surrounding structures. Obstructive sinusitis, mucocele formation, and intrusion on the intracranial and orbital spaces with resultant maladies have all been reported in association with paranasal sinus osteomas. Treatment is by surgical excision, frequently possible via endoscopic techniques, although some of the more lateral frontal sinus lesions are more easily removed via an osteoplastic or combined approach. It is often necessary to perform a Draf II or III, or an endoscopic modified Lothrop procedure, to gain adequate endoscopic exposure. A surgeon should expect and be prepared to manage periorbital and dural injuries, as they are occasionally unavoidable when removing these lesions via either endoscopic or external approaches.

Fibrous dysplasia and ossifying fibroma are other fibro-osseous lesions found in the paranasal sinuses. Fibrous dysplasia affects children and characteristically "burns out" during puberty. It is deforming but not destructive and appears as a ground glass density on plain film radiograph or CT. In the polyostotic form, it is associated with McCune-Albright syndrome. A conservative treatment strategy is recommended, reserving surgical intervention for symptomatic lesions. Ossifying fibroma is more serious. Appearing as a well-circumscribed lesion with an eggshell-thin wall and a hypodense center, OF can be locally destructive and should be aggressively and completely excised.

Acknowledgements

The authors would like to thank Walter Bell, MD, for the histologic photomicrograph.

References

[1] Summers LE, Mascott CR, Tompkins JR, et al. Frontal sinus osteoma associated with cerebral abscess formation: a case report. Surg Neurol 2001;55(4):235–9.
[2] Chen C, Selva D, Wormald PJ. Endoscopic modified Lothrop procedure: an alternative for frontal osteoma excision. Rhinology 2004;42(4):239–43.
[3] Johnson D, Tan L. Intraparenchymal tension pneumatocele complicating frontal sinus osteoma: case report. Neurosurgery 2002;50(4):878–9 [discussion: 880].
[4] Moretti A, Croce A, Leone O, et al. Osteoma of maxillary sinus: case report. Acta Otorhinolaryngol Ital 2004;24(4):219–22.
[5] Naraghi M, Kashfi A. Endonasal endoscopic resection of ethmoido-orbital osteoma compressing the optic nerve. Am J Otolaryngol 2003;24(6):408–12.
[6] Osma U, Yaldiz M, Tekin M, et al. Giant ethmoid osteoma with orbital extension presenting with epiphora. Rhinology 2003;41(2):122–4.

[7] Sayan NB, Ucok C, Karasu HA, et al. Peripheral osteoma of the oral and maxillofacial region: a study of 35 new cases. J Oral Maxillofac Surg 2002;60(11):1299–301.

[8] Schick B, Steigerwald C, el Rahman el Tahan A, et al. The role of endonasal surgery in the management of frontoethmoidal osteomas. Rhinology 2001;39(2):66–70.

[9] Vowles RH, Bleach NR. Frontoethmoid osteoma. Ann Otol Rhinol Laryngol 1999;108(5): 522–4.

[10] Mahabir RC, Szymczak A, Sutherland GR. Intracerebral pneumatocele presenting after air travel. J Neurosurg 2004;101(2):340–2.

[11] Sell S. Stem cell origin of cancer and differentiation therapy. Crit Rev Oncol Hematol 2004; 51(1):1–28.

[12] Rawlins AG. Osteoma of the maxillary sinus. Annals of Otol Rhinol Laryngol 1938;47: 735–53.

[13] Nabeshima K, Marutsuka K, Shimao Y, et al. Osteoma of the frontal sinus complicated by intracranial mucocele. Pathol Int 2003;53(4):227–30.

[14] Gezici AR, Okay O, Ergun R, et al. Rare intracranial manifestations of frontal osteomas. Acta Neurochir (Wien) 2004;146(4):393–6 [discussion: 396].

[15] Tsai CJ, Ho CY, Lin CZ. A huge osteoma of paranasal sinuses with intraorbital extension presenting as diplopia. J Chin Med Assoc 2003;66(7):433–5.

[16] Tsai TL, Ho CY, Guo YC, et al. Fibrous dysplasia of the ethmoid sinus. J Chin Med Assoc 2003;66(2):131–3.

[17] Akay KM, Onguru O, Sirin S, et al. Association of paranasal sinus osteoma and intracranial mucocele–two case reports. Neurol Med Chir (Tokyo) 2004;44(4):201–4.

[18] Koyuncu M, Belet U, Sesen T, et al. Huge osteoma of the frontoethmoidal sinus with secondary brain abscess. Auris Nasus Larynx 2000;27(3):285–7.

[19] London SD, Schlosser RJ, Gross CW. Endoscopic management of benign sinonasal tumors: a decade of experience. Am J Rhinol 2002;16(4):221–7.

[20] Roca B, Casado O, Borras JM, et al. Frontal brain abscess due to Streptococcus pneumoniae associated with an osteoma. Int J Infect Dis 2004;8(3):193.

[21] Rappaport JM, Attia EL. Pneumocephalus in frontal sinus osteoma: a case report. J Otolaryngol 1994;23(6):430–6.

[22] Selva D, Chen C, Wormald PJ. Frontoethmoidal osteoma: a stereotactic-assisted sino-orbital approach. Ophthal Plast Reconstr Surg 2003;19(3):237–8.

[23] Lindman JT, Sillers MJ. Operative trephination for non-acute frontal sinus disease. Operative Techniques in Otolaryngology–Head and Neck Surgery 2004;15(1):67–70.

[24] Buch B, Noffke C, de Kock S. Gardner's syndrome–the importance of early diagnosis: a case report and a review. SADJ 2001;56(5):242–5.

[25] MacDonald-Jankowski DS. Fibro-osseous lesions of the face and jaws. Clin Radiol 2004; 59(1):11–25.

ELSEVIER
SAUNDERS

Otolaryngol Clin N Am
39 (2006) 601–617

OTOLARYNGOLOGIC
CLINICS
OF NORTH AMERICA

Benign Sinonasal Neoplasms: A Focus on Inverting Papilloma

Christopher T. Melroy, MD, Brent A. Senior, MD*

Department of Otolaryngology–Head and Neck Surgery, University of North Carolina Hospitals, 101 Manning Drive, CB #7070, Chapel Hill, NC 27514, USA

Benign tumors of the sinonasal tract are a histologically diverse group of neoplasms that may have similar clinical presentations. When symptomatic, they generally present because of a mass effect and perturbation of surrounding normal structures. Nasal airway obstruction, epistaxis, epiphora, rhinorrhea, and recurrent sinusitis are common presenting symptoms. Tumors also may be asymptomatic; these generally present as incidental findings on radiographic imaging performed for nonrhinologic purposes. Although the differential diagnosis of such a lesion may be narrowed by historical, endoscopic, and radiographic information at the time of presentation, the diagnosis rests on pathologic analysis of a biopsy specimen.

These tumors can be divided into several groups: fibro–osseous (osteoma, chondroma, ossifying fibroma, and fibrous dysplasia), neural-related (schwannoma, neurofibroma, and meningioma), hamartomatous (respiratory epithelial adenomatoid hamartoma) and odontogenic (ameloblastoma, and calcifying epithelial tumor of Pindborg), vascular (hemangioma, hemangiopericytoma, juvenile nasopharyngeal angiofibroma, and pyogenic granuloma), and inverted papilloma.

Fibro–osseous tumors

Osteoma is the most common benign sinonasal tumor, and it has been reported to be seen on 1% of routine sinus radiographs, most commonly localized to the frontal sinus [1]. These tumors are slow growing and well circumscribed, with symptoms generally attributable to obstruction of the drainage pathway of nearby sinuses. When symptoms are present, the symptom complex most commonly includes frontal pain and headache [2,3]. On

---

* Corresponding author.
E-mail address: bsenior@med.unc.edu (B.A. Senior).

0030-6665/06/$ - see front matter © 2006 Elsevier Inc. All rights reserved.
doi:10.1016/j.otc.2006.01.005

endoscopy, they appear as firm masses with a smooth mucosal covering (Figs. 1,2). Their management has been documented, and it depends on their location, rate of growth, symptoms, and effect on surrounding structures [4]. Gardner's syndrome is an autosomal-dominant condition consisting of osteomas (usually multiple), soft tissue tumors (such as epidermal inclusion cysts or subcutaneous fibrous tumors), and polyposis of the colon. This triad of symptoms should be remembered by otolaryngologists, and should prompt gastroenterology referral if this is suspected, as malignant degeneration of these colonic polyps will occur in 40% of patients [3].

Differentiation between ossifying fibroma and fibrous dysplasia is important, as the management of these benign fibro–osseous tumors may differ. Radiographically, fibrous dysplasia characteristically has a ground glass appearance on CT images. It generally presents in younger patients (children and adolescents), and its growth rate may decrease or stop after puberty. Because of this, the management of fibrous dysplasia of the sinonasal cavity is generally expectant or conservative [5]. Again, familiarity with systemic syndromes is essential to the practice of rhinology. McCune-Albright's syndrome is a disseminated form of polyostotic fibrous dysplasia that also manifests with precocious puberty, early skeletal bone maturation, and abnormal skin pigmentation [6,7].

Ossifying fibroma, on the other hand, has a more aggressive growth pattern and can exhibit rapid bony erosion and become locally destructive. Although this tumor is found most commonly in the mandible, the sinonasal counterparts tend to be more destructive [8]. The management pattern of ossifying fibroma should reflect the nature of this tumor, and resection generally is recommended early in the disease process. Endoscopic resection of these tumors may be feasible but is associated with a higher recurrence rate than other benign tumors [5].

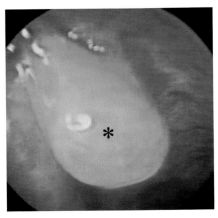

Fig. 1. An endoscopic, endonasal view of an osteoma reveals a firm lesion (*) with a normal mucosal covering.

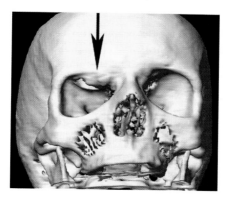

Fig. 2. Three-dimensional reconstruction of a sinus CT of a patient with an osteoma (*arrow*) of anterior table of the frontal sinus. This view demonstrates the effect of the tumor on the volume of the globe. This outward expansion caused vision changes and diplopia, and the internal growth of the osteoma resulted in a frontal sinus mucocele.

Other benign tumors

Neural-related tumors include meningiomas, schwannomas, and neurofibromas. Meningiomas are encountered infrequently in the nose and paranasal sinuses and arise from ectopic arachnoid tissue. Their growth is generally expansile in nature, and can be difficult at times to differentiate from intracranial meningioma. The skull base is generally intact in sinonasal cases, and the bowing of bone is generally in a direction toward the skull base [9]. Schwannomas generally present along the nasal septum as they arise from branches of the trigeminal nerve [10], but they can present along on peripheral nerves (Fig. 3). Similarly, neurofibromas can arise from peripheral nerves in the sinonasal cavity; differential diagnosis of these neoplasms relies on pathologic analysis of the tumor.

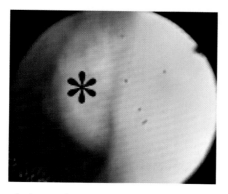

Fig. 3. Endoscopic view depicts a schwannoma (*) arising from the superior turbinate in the sphenoethmoidal recess.

Hamartomatous lesions of the sinonasal tract are tumors composed of cells that, at some point during development, were a normal part of the local anatomy. They include respiratory epithelial adenomatoid hamartoma (REAH) and odontogenic tumors. The two hamartomas of odontogenic origin primarily seen in this area are ameloblastoma and the calcifying epithelial tumor of Pindborg. Twenty percent of all ameloblastomas arise in the maxilla, and the sinuses generally are involved after secondary growth into these air-containing spaces (Fig. 4) [11]. Pindborg's tumors are much rarer and can present clinically in a fashion similar to ameloblastoma.

Juvenile nasopharyngeal angiofibroma (JNA) is seen in males and generally presents in the second decade of life with nasal airway obstruction and epistaxis. This is a firm, well-encapsulated tumor that usually arises near the sphenopalatine foramen near the posterior attachment of the middle turbinate. Its growth may lead to a dumbbell-shaped tumor with one lobe growing into the nasopharynx and the other toward the pterygopalatine fossa. Resection of this tumor may involve preoperative embolization, and endoscopic techniques frequently are employed [12]. Other vascular benign neoplasms of the sinonasal tract include hemangiomas, hemangiopericytomas, and pyogenic granulomas. A review of these and other tumors are beyond the scope of this article.

Inverted papilloma

Inverted papilloma (IP) is a distinct clinical and pathological entity with a long and rich history. It is characterized best by its local invasion, tendency for recurrence, and association with malignancy.

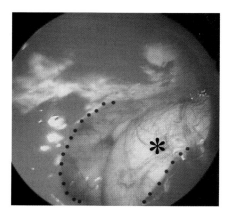

Fig. 4. Endoscopic view demonstrates an ameloblastoma that extended into the maxillary sinus. A large middle meatal antrostomy was made (*detailed with dotted line*), and a 70° endoscope was directed toward the inferior wall allowed exposure to the tumor (*).

Historical perspective

In 1854, Ward was the first to document and detail the occurrence of papilloma in the sinonasal cavity [13]. Soon after this, Biliroth described two papillomatous growths within the nasal cavity and deemed them "villiform cancers" in 1855 [14]. Hoppman also gained experience with these tumors, and, in 1883, subcategorized these into hard and soft papillomas based on the texture of their epithelial lining [15]. It was Reingertz in 1935, however, who histologically described the epithelium of this tumor and noted that it inverted into the underlying connective tissue [16]. Since that time, this tumor, which shows histological inversion of the epithelium, has been called a myriad of descriptive terms, including: inverting papilloma, inverted papilloma, epithelial papilloma, papillary sinusitis, Schneiderian papilloma, inverted Schneiderian papilloma, soft papilloma, transitional cell papilloma, cylindrical cell carcinoma, polyp with inverting metaplasia, and benign transitional cell growth [17]. This, in part, reflects the initial lack of understanding of this tumor by clinicians and pathologists.

The efforts of Hyams served to remedy this issue. In 1971, Hyams reviewed 315 cases on papillomas from the nose and paranasal sinuses at the Armed Forces Institute of Pathology [18]. The report of these findings served to solidify the terminology and pathology of inverting papillomas, thus making clinicians and pathologists aware that this is a distinct and single clinicopathological entity. This report subdivided sinonasal papillomas into inverted, fungiform, and cylindrical cell types, which some feel simply reflects the local environment of the tumor [19].

Pathology

Grossly, the tumor appears exophytic and polypoid, yet it appears more vascular than an inflammatory polyp (Fig. 5). The tumor may be gray to pink and often has frond-like projections that extend from the main bulk of the specimen [17]. Although it may fill the nasal cavity to a variable degree, the site of localization to the native mucosa is often a discrete pedicle-like connection. Depending on its size and extent, the tumor may rest against other mucosa within the nasal cavity; similarly, it may occupy a sinus and rest against its mucosa. When IP occupies such an area without arising from it, the tumor bulk simply rests on the nearby mucosa, a mucosa that remains normal without evidence of invasion or any change caused by the nearby tumor.

IP gets the moniker inverted from the histologic appearance of the neoplastic epithelium. Microscopically, the epithelium of the IP is distinct from the respiratory (pseudostratified ciliated columnar) mucosa of the sinonasal cavity, and the epithelial cell may be squamous, transitional, or respiratory [17]. This epithelium is proliferative and is thickened compared with the surrounding normal epithelium and lacks mucus-secreting cells and eosinophils [20]. The nuclear to cytoplasm ratio is normal, and there are few (less than

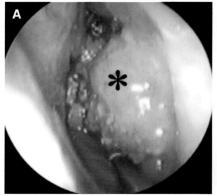
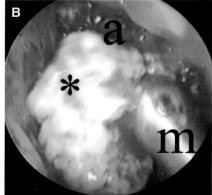

Fig. 5. (*A*) Intraoperative photographs of the right anterior nasal cavity reveal inverting papilloma (*), which at first inspection appears to emanate from the nasal septum. (*B*) A microdebrider (**m**) is used to manipulate the tumor and reveal normal underlying mucosa. The
microdebrider is used to debulk tumor and helped to more clearly define the tumor attachment
(**a**) to the lateral nasal wall in the middle meatus.

two) mitotic figures per high-powered field. Squamous metaplasia may occur, and the cells may become hyperkeratotic, with an overlying thin layer
of keratin on the smooth surface of the tumor. The orderly maturation of
cells from the basal layer outward is maintained. When viewed from low
power, the inverting, endophytic nature of the epithelium is seen best and
is markedly different from the histologically exophytic appearance of common papillomas. Also, there is no koilocytosis, which is present in common
papillomas and would appear as vacuolization of cells near the surface.

The epithelium rests upon an intact basement membrane that is not invaded or interrupted by the overlying cells. It is not thickened and does
not show any inflammatory changes. Microscopically, the epithelial layer in-
vaginates into the underlying (subepithelial) stroma, which consists of
a loose connective tissue without signs of desmoplasia [21] (Figs. 6, 7).

The diagnosis of IP depends on a tissue biopsy, which generally is taken
in a clinical setting before definitive treatment. The cytologic appearance of
the tumor (obtained by a touch preparation) has been shown to correlate
with the histologic findings of IP, but its clinical use had not been adopted
widely [22].

Etiology

There have been no widely accepted causative factors associated with IP.
It is felt that the entire Schneiderian membrane (the embryologic origin of
the mucous membranes of the sinonasal cavity) is at risk for the development of this epithelial neoplasm, and this eponym has persisted as a descriptor of IP [23]. The role of allergy has been discounted because of the lack of

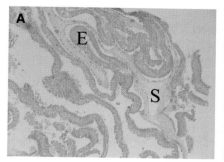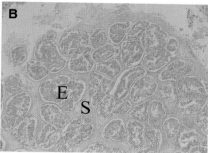

Fig. 6. (*A*) Tubular fronds of epithelium (*E*) invert into the underlying stroma (*S*). Hematoxylin and eosin stained sections of inverted papilloma are shown at low power. (*B*) The representative section was cut perpendicular to the long axis of these fronds, so multiple cross-sections of the epithelial fronds (*E*) are seen inverting into the stroma (*S*). Hematoxylin and eosin stained sections of inverted papilloma are shown at low power.

a personal history of allergic rhinitis in patients who develop IP. Chronic rhinosinusitis also has been presented as a possible etiologic factor, as this generally is associated temporally with IP [24]. It has been elucidated that the rhinosinusitis seen in patients with IP is secondary to alteration of the sinuses' natural drainage pathways by tumor. No association between to-bacco products or alcohol use has been found. Although environmental ex-posures have been known to predispose individuals to sinonasal carcinomas, there has been no link established between this and IP.

A viral etiology for IP has been sought, likely because of the association between common papillomas and the human papillomavirus (HPV) [25]. Electron microscopy has failed to show ultrastructural evidence of viral par-ticles in IP [26,27], and immunohistochemical techniques have not shown HPV antigens in IP [28,29]. Using in situ hybridization techniques, however,

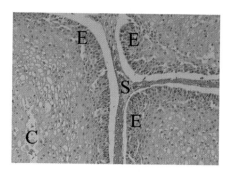

Fig. 7. Three epithelial fronds (*E*) are seen invaginating into the stroma (*S*). The core (*C*) of these fronds is fibrovascular. Note the orderly organization of the epithelial cells from the basal layer to the surface and the lack of mitotic figures. Hematoxylin and eosin stained sections of inverted papilloma are shown at high power.

HPV DNA has been found in IP specimens and is similar to that in HPV types 6 and 11 [30,31]. Still, the fact that HPV DNA has been found in these lesions is not enough to support a viral etiology for IP. Some, however, suggest HPV may be implicated in cases with multi-centric disease, dysplasia, malignancy, and the garden-variety tumor [32].

Clinical aspects of inverting papilloma

The incidence of IP has been documented at 0.2 [33] to 0.6 [34] cases per 100,000 people per year. It comprises 0.5% to 4% of primary nasal tumors [20] and is 1/25 as frequent as inflammatory polyps [35]. Weissler and colleagues [19] have reported the largest single report on their 35-year experience with IP that included 223 cases. The symptom complex reported by this group parallels that of other investigators and includes unilateral nasal obstruction (58%), epistaxis (17%), nasal drainage (14%), bilateral nasal obstruction (12%), nasal mass (9%), and sinusitis (9%). Other common presenting symptoms include headache, diplopia, facial numbness, facial swelling, and anosmia [20,36]. In a review of several large case series, the average time patients experienced these symptoms ranged from 27 to 66 months [20,37]. This surprising number is a reflection of the relatively innocuous and very nonspecific symptom complex experienced by this patient group. These symptoms overlap with a myriad of other conditions including allergy, chronic rhinosinusitis, and migraine.

Classically, IP has a predilection for males with a male:female ratio of 3:1. There is no side predilection, and cases are usually unilateral. Bilateral lesions are seen in 4.9% of patients [14]. There is no notable race predilection, as the rates mimic that of the standard population [19]. In a collection of 522 patients from five different studies, the average age was 54.3 years at the time of treatment [19,20,36,37,38], and it generally is reported to be most common in the fifth and sixth decades of life [39].

Krouse reviewed and summarized the published experiences with IP from 1967 to 1997. The primary sites of IP origin were documented including the lateral nasal wall (82%), maxillary sinus (53.9%), ethmoid sinus (31.6%), septum (9.9%), frontal sinus (6.5%), and the sphenoid sinus (3.9%) [14,40].

Radiographic findings

Although there are classic radiographic findings associated with IP, there are no pathognomonic findings of IP on imaging [41,42]. There is, however, still information to be obtained from these studies that can assist in the diagnosis and operative management [43]. CT and MRI are the common modalities used to evaluate IP. In a review of the literature, CT is the most widely performed study, and this better details bony anatomy. From a diagnostic standpoint, inverted papilloma is associated with bony changes. The most common bony finding is bowing of the bones near the soft tissue mass. Tumors that extend into the maxillary sinus cause widening of the infundibulum on CT and make the uncinate process difficult to discern [41].

There is a classic association of IP with the term bony erosion. From a clinical perspective, this term connotes aggressive invasion of normal structures and usually is reserved for describing malignancies. The mass effect from IP is a slow and constant force on the surrounding mucosal and bony structures that can cause the affected bone to remodel. This bony remodeling is a better descriptor of the bony changes seen on CT [41], and it most commonly is seen at the medial wall of the maxillary sinus followed by the lamina papyracea [20]. Published series show a wide range of this finding, from 7% to 50% [17].

It has been postulated that the skull base has a different radiographic appearance in response to IP than that of other sinonasal bones. In the setting of IP near the floor of the anterior or middle cranial fossa, the bones of the skull base tend to resemble bone destruction. Unlike the relatively plastic facial bones, it is proposed that the skull base has a limited response to pressure; instead of remodeling, they just appear to erode and radiologically mimic malignancy [41,44] Also, because of the thin and sieve-like nature of the cribriform plate, intracranial extension can occur even without dramatic bony changes on imaging [45].

The association of CT evidence of bony erosion with malignancy in IP is also debated; one study [46] reports this finding in 100% of malignant specimen, while another shows 0% [47]. A similar scenario is seen with MRI and the detection of an IP-associated malignancy; there are no features present on MRI that differentiate IP from IP with malignancy or squamous cell carcinoma alone [45].

Sukenik et al [48] compared CT imaging with intraoperative nasal endoscopy to discern the ability of each to evaluate tumor extent. The sensitivity of each was identical at 69%, but the specificity of endoscopy exceeded that of CT (68% versus 20%). Endoscopy also had a better positive predictive value (55% versus 36%) and negative predictive value (91% versus 64%). Although both modalities seem to exaggerate the extent of disease, the presence of a normal intraoperative endoscopy is superior to CT in determining the extent of mucosa removal.

Contrasted CT may show slight enhancement of IP, and calcifications may be present. This is a nonspecific finding, but IP and esthesioneuroblastomas are the two most common nasal tumors associated with intralesional calcification [41].

Compared with CT, MRI better characterizes soft tissue structures. In MRI, IP is hypodense to isodense on T1-weighted images and isodense to hyperdense on T2-weighted images. The mass slightly enhances with contrast and appears nonhomogeneous. The biggest advantage of MRI in the radiographic analysis of IP is differentiating tumor soft tissue from inspissated mucus, as these are hyperintense on T2-weighted images [41,45].

Association with carcinoma

An association between IP and squamous cell carcinoma (SCCa) exists; however, the exact details of this relationship are the matter of some controversy. In addition to the propensity of IP to cause local destruction, it is the association with malignancy that has driven therapy for these tumors. In his analysis of 30 years of published reports, Krouse documents the finding of carcinoma in 9.1% of all patients [14].

SCCa may present in the setting of IP in three different scenarios. First, a patient may have an inverting papilloma with small foci of SCCa within it. Also, some patients present with discrete and separate sinonasal tumors—both IP and SCCa at the same time—without evidence that the malignancy arose from the IP. Both of these scenarios are deemed synchronous, but it is not clear how these are related. The third entity is the metachronous malignancy, one that manifests in the area of a prior IP resection well after the time of primary tumor removal [17]. In many reports of malignancy in the setting of IP, these details are not included in the discussion of the tumor, which hinders better characterization.

It has been postulated that synchronous IP and SCCa share a common cellular lineage. Lawson suggests a common unstable or metaplastic epithelium gives rise to these two distinct pathologic entities that are related but remain separate [49]. The true relation is not known.

Metachronous carcinoma is much less common that its synchronous counterparts. Of the 233 patients, Weissler and colleagues [19] reported 11 malignancies, four of which were metachronous. Of 87 patients, Lawson reported five malignancies, one of which was metachronous [17]. Many authors consider IP to be a premalignant tumor because of these findings [14]. There have been case series and isolated presentations to solidify this thought. Vrabec followed an individual for 3 years with repeated biopsy of an initially benign IP. Over this time period, atypia developed and progressed to the point of SCCa, a finding reaffirmed by other studies [50,51].

There are no documented pathologic or clinical findings in IP associated with the future development of SCCa. Wormald suggests malignant disease is associated with bilateral IP, hyperkeratosis, greater than two mitotic figures per high-powered field, and presence of plasma cells [52]. In contrast, Suh and colleagues reported that atypical features in benign IP do not predict future development of carcinoma or recurrence of IP [53]. Also, the number of recurrences of IP does not correlate with the propensity for malignancy.

The malignancy issue (along with local destruction and recurrence) drives the treatment paradigm of standard IP. Whether IP is a true premalignant lesion remains a matter of debate.

Treatment regimens and rates of recurrence

Since the publication of Hyams in 1971, there has been an increased understanding and awareness of inverting papilloma. With the standardization of reporting and increasing communication between clinicians, the management algorithm for IP has evolved.

Early surgical experiences with IP were fraught with high recurrence rates. These procedures, which had a curative intent, generally used the transnasal (closed) approach. Illumination was provided by a headlight (at best), and local tumor removal was attempted by local, simple resections that mimicked polypectomies [52]. An outcome analysis dealing with this type of procedure was published in 1971 and revealed a staggering recurrence rate of 71% [54].

As the understanding of IP progressed, the standard surgical approach became more aggressive. External procedures such as the Caldwell-Luc and external ethmoidectomy provided increase access to the sinonasal cavity. Open procedures with a lateral rhinotomy or midface degloving approaches allowed for increased visualization of the tumor bed and more complete resections than any of the prior methods, and most resections involved some form of maxillectomy.

In Weissler's 35-year review [19], treatment was subdivided into transnasal, external, and open. They noted the recurrence rate varied inversely with the extent of the procedure and was 71% for intranasal procedures, 56% for external procedures (Caldwell-Luc or some variation of external ethmoidectomy), and 29% for open procedures (lateral rhinotomy or midface degloving). In light of these recurrence rates, this study proposed the lateral rhinotomy approach as the standard of care for surgical treatment of inverting papilloma.

These recommendations were accepted widely by the surgical community, and open exposure, coupled with en bloc resections (usually involving some sort of maxillectomy), was performed routinely for extirpation of disease. The complication rate was acceptable and included ozena, diplopia, epiphora, nasal stenosis, bleeding, and death. As proposed, open management of IP had become the accepted and widely practiced standard of care. Numerous presentations of case series documented its effectiveness [51].

While investigating their experiences over a 15 year period, Lawson and colleagues [17] had a special patient population treated without an open approach that had recurrence rates similar to their standard resections. Ten patients with tumors limited to the inferior or middle meatus with minimal maxillary and ethmoid sinus involvement were treated by transnasal or transantral sphenoethmoidectomy. This procedure was chosen over the classic lateral rhinotomy and midface degloving approaches, as these patients were either not candidates for general anesthesia or had an initial erroneous biopsy specimen. The recurrence rate for these patients (10%) mirrored that of the 75 patients they treated with the classic open approach (9%). This and other studies suggested that, in certain clinical situations where tumor extent is limited, a more conservative approach to resection is a viable option for managing IP [17].

This concept was extrapolated into the endoscopic realm. In the mid-1980s, endoscopic sinus surgery was popularized, and the initial experience was to diagnose and treat inflammatory disorders of the nose and paranasal sinuses. As the familiarity with this new technique grew, so did the applications of endoscopic endonasal surgery. Its use in the surgical management of IP began as an extension of the ideals of Lawson and colleagues; certain tumors with limited extent could be treated successfully by a modality that was conservative and avoided an open approach. Endoscopic management fit this tenet, and Waitz and Wigand were the first to detail a case series on endoscopically treated patients. They noted a recurrence rate of this method similar to the more classic open approach (17% versus 19%) [55], and this was reaffirmed by other investigators also [56,57].

In all of the studies, it was detailed explicitly that endoscopic management was reserved for treating limited and easily accessible tumors. These generally were confined to the lateral nasal wall with possible minimal extension into the anterior ethmoid sinus. Because of this, the comparison of results of endoscopic versus open management was confounded by selection bias. The recurrence rates of endoscopic management of straightforward tumors were being compared with that of open management of more extensive and complex tumors. No widely accepted staging system could be used to standardize reporting [58].

As the experience with endoscopic sinus surgery for managing inflammatory conditions extended to tumor resection, surgeons had greater confidence in the management of more complex benign sinonasal tumors. First, more bulky tumors were addressed endoscopically. In situations where a large nasal IP fills the nasal cavity but is only physically associated with a small mucosal area, debulking of most the tumor with a microdebrider while retaining its site of attachment is of import (Fig. 5). This allows a better survey of the sinonasal cavity and allows better characterization of the attachment of the IP to the native nasal mucosa. It also serves to direct therapy to the specific area of pathology.

The endoscopic management of the bony architecture surrounding IP also evolved as more extensive tumors were addressed. Groups have discussed the resection of underlying bone when possible [38] and drilling the surface of the bone when not possible. As more extensive tumors were addressed in more sites than just the lateral nasal wall and the anterior ethmoid sinus, however, more invasive endoscopic procedures have been characterized. The goal of these procedures is to provide adequate exposure for resection and postoperative surveillance of the tumor bed.

Endoscopic techniques also have been applied to management of IP of the maxillary sinus. One distinct advantage of endoscopic approaches is that they also may incorporate adjunctive open procedures such as trephination and Caldwell-Luc to improve access or exposure [38]. Endoscopic management of IP of the maxillary sinus necessitates improved visualization of the sinus cavity, as even a 70° scope can fail to allow visualization of the entire cavity. Therefore, a maxillary canine fossa puncture is essential to the use of endoscopy to manage maxillary sinus IP. This puncture site allows the introduction of the endoscope to allow total visualization when working transnasally and allows the passage of instrumentation while the endoscope is transnasal.

For tumors of the posterior wall of the maxillary sinus, a wide middle meatal antrostomy with removal of bone and mucosa flush to the posterior wall and roof of the maxillary sinus allows excellent exposure. Instrumentation introduced from a canine fossa puncture increases access. For involvement of the floor, anterior, lateral, or medial walls of the maxillary sinus, a form of endoscopic medial maxillectomy is needed. Wormald and colleagues [52] and Sadeghi and colleagues [59] give excellent detailed descriptions of the procedure, the end result of which removes the medial portion of the maxillary sinus and lateral nasal wall while retaining the medial buttress of the maxilla. Sadeghi and colleagues emphasized that the transnasal endoscopic medial maxillectomy is minimally invasive and allows the resection of tumor as an en bloc specimen. They feel this is more oncologically sound than endoscopic piecemeal removal, which they tout as "basically a form of extended sinus surgery, not a medial maxillectomy" [59].

IP of the frontal sinus and frontal recess has the potential to be managed endoscopically; however, careful patient and case selection is key to success. At best, nasal endoscopy provides limited access to the frontal sinus, and management of a neoplasm in this area is difficult [4]. The endoscopic modified Lothrop procedure [60] has been implemented successfully in selected cases of IP of the frontal sinus and frontal recess. In unilateral disease, operating on the uninvolved frontal sinus predisposes the patient to the morbidity of the surgery; however, this is acceptable, as it allows margins to be assessed better intraoperatively and allows improved tumor surveillance postoperatively [52]. In IP involving the lateral frontal sinus, endoscopic resection is not encouraged if the anatomy precludes adequate access. In these cases, osteoplastic flap without obliteration is encouraged. No obliteration is recommended so the primary site may be followed better radiographically and endoscopically. Creating a wide frontal sinusotomy at the time of tumor removal increases visualization for surveillance in the postoperative period [56].

In Krouse's review of 30 years of published data on 1426 patients, the recurrence rates of IP in multiple types of procedures were analyzed. For the analysis of recurrence data, he categorized the surgical approaches of this period into four groups: nonendoscopic intranasal, conservative (Caldwell-Luc, transnasal, and transantral procedures short of an en bloc resection), aggressive (en bloc resection of tumor by means of midface degloving, lateral rhinotomy, or Weber-Ferguson incision), and endoscopic (including all endoscopic approaches). The recurrence rates for these groups were 67.3%, 44.0%, 18.0%, and 11.8%, respectively (Table 1). There was no statistical difference between the recurrence rates of the aggressive and endoscopic groups [14].

Table 1
Recurrence rates [14]

Treatment type	Percent recurrence
Intranasal (without endoscopy)	67.3
Conservative (Caldwell-Luc, external ethmoidectomy procedures)	44.0
Aggressive (lateral rhinotomy, midface degloving, maxillectomy)	18.0
Endoscopic and extended endoscopic	11.8

As previously stated, there is a selection bias that confounds these data. In the current era, only certain tumors are treated endoscopically, and a comparison of the recurrence rate of this group must take this into account. In an effort to standardize disease reporting and communication between investigators, Krouse has developed a staging system for IP. This is not the first staging system proposed for IP, but it does take into account salient clinical factors that are germane to the description of the disease process. The factors that determine a patient's stage are also important factors in the selection of a surgical approach, and they include extent of disease, location of disease, and the presence of malignancy. This four-stage system (Box 1) mimics that of the T staging system of the American Joint Committee on Cancer [58]. T1 lesions can be treated with endoscopic techniques without much resection of bone; T2 tumors are also accessible with endoscopic techniques but require some removal of bony structures. T3 lesions have the potential to be managed endoscopically if adequate visualization can be achieved; similarly, an open procedure with medial maxillectomy could be used to manage this type of IP. Lastly, an open surgical approach is recommended for T4 tumors to provide maximal exposure [14].

The management algorithm of IP has come full-circle and has returned to transnasal approaches, although current transnasal techniques are performed under endoscopic visualization. Endoscopy and powered instrumentation allow more extensive transnasal surgery to be done with better tumor identification and localization. As the sites of tumor involvement are visualized better, a more directed resection is possible, incurring less trauma to the

---

Box 1. Krouse staging system for inverting papilloma [58]

T1—Tumor isolated to one area of the nasal cavity without extension to paranasal sinuses.

T2—Tumor involves medial wall of maxillary sinus, ethmoid sinuses, and/or osteomeatal complex

T3—Tumor involves the superior, inferior, posterior, anterior, or lateral walls of the maxillary sinus; frontal sinus; or sphenoid sinus.

T4—Tumor with extrasinonasal extent or malignancy

surrounding mucosa and anatomic structures. These concepts apply some principles of functional endoscopic sinus surgery to the management of IP.

Summary

Benign sinonasal neoplasms are a pathologic and clinically varied group of tumors. Inverting papilloma is a notable member of this group, and it is renowned for its high rate of recurrence, its ability to cause local destruction, and its association with malignancy. This article aimed to familiarize the clinician with all the practical aspects of inverting papilloma and its management. The treatment algorithm for this tumor has undergone a complex evolution that continues today.

References

[1] Mehta B, Grewal G. Osteoma of the paranasal sinuses along with a case of orbito–ethmoid osteoma. J Laryngol Otol 1963;17:601.

[2] Atallah N, Jay M. Osteomas of the paranasal sinuses. J Laryngol Otol 1981;95:291.

[3] Smith M, Calcaterra T. Frontal sinus osteoma. Ann Otol Rhinol Laryngol 1989;98:896.

[4] Senior B, Lanza D. Benign lesions of the frontal sinus. Otolaryngol Clin North Am 2001; 34(1):253–67.

[5] London SD, Schlosser RJ, Gross CW. Endoscopic management of benign sinonasal tumors: a decade of experience. Am J Rhinol 2002;16(4):221–7.

[6] Lichtenstein L. Polyostotic fibrous dysplasia. Arch Surg 1938;36:874–98.

[7] Verdaguer JM, Lobo D, Garcia-Berrocal JR, et al. Radiology quiz case 4. McCune-Albright syndrome. Arch Otolaryngol Head Neck Surg 2005;131(2):181–5.

[8] Vaidya AM, Chow JM, Goldberg K, et al. Juvenile aggressive ossifying fibroma presenting as en ethmoid sinus mucocele. Otolaryngol Head Neck Surg 1998;119(6):665–8.

[9] Daneshi A, Asghari A, Bahramy E. Primary meningioma of the ethmoid sinus: a case report. Ear Nose Throat J 2003;82(4):310–1.

[10] Shinohara K, Hashimoto K, Yamashita M, et al. Schwannoma of the nasal septum removed with endoscopic surgery. Otolaryngol Head Neck Surg 2005;132(6):963–4.

[11] Shinohara K, Hashimoto K, Yamashita M, et al. Primary sinonasal ameloblastoma. APMIS 2005;113(2):148–50.

[12] Pryor SG, Moore EJ, Kasperbauer JL. Endoscopic versus traditional approaches for excision of juvenile nasopharyngeal angiofibromas. Laryngoscope 2005;115(7):1201–7.

[13] Ward N. A mirror of the practice of medicine and surgery in the hospitals of London. London Hospital Lancet 1854;2:480–2.

[14] Krouse JH. Endoscopic treatment of inverted papilloma: safety and efficacy. Am J Otolaryngol 2001;22(2):87–99.

[15] Hoppmann CM. Die Papillaren Geschwulste der Nasenshleimhaut. Virchows Archives of Pathologic Anatomy 1883;93:213–58.

[16] Ringertz N. Pathology of malignant tumors arising in nasal and paranasal cavities and maxilla. Acta Otolaryngol 1938;27:31–42 [suppl].

[17] Lawson W, Le Benger J, Som P, et al. Inverted papilloma: an analysis of 87 cases. Laryngoscope 1989;99(11):1117–24.

[18] Hyams VJ. Papillomas of the nasal cavity and paranasal sinuses: a clinicopathological study of 315 cases. Ann Otol Rhinol Laryngol 1971;80(2):192–206.

[19] Weissler MC, Montgomery WW, Montgomery SK, et al. Inverted papilloma. Ann Otol Rhinol Laryngol 1986;95:215–21.

[20] Vrabec DP. The inverted Schneiderian papilloma: a 25-year study. Laryngoscope 1994;104: 582–605.

[21] Calhoun K, Kumar D, Weiss R. Basic head and neck pathology. Rochester (MN): Custom Printing; 1995.

[22] Gould VE, Manosca F, Reddy VB, et al. Cytologic-histologic correlations in the diagnosis of inverted sinonasal papilloma. Diagn Cytopathol 2004;30(3):201–7.

[23] Stammberger L. New aspects of aetiology and mopthology of the inverting papilloma. Laryngol Rhinol Otol (Stuttg) 1983;62:249–55.

[24] Kramer R, Som JL. True papilloma of the nasal cavity. Arch Otolaryngol 1935;22:22–43.

[25] Frenkiel S, Mongiardo FD, Tewfik TL, et al. Viral implications in the formation of multi-centric inverting papilloma. J Otolaryngol 1994;23(6):419–22.

[26] Gaito RA, Gaylord WH, Hilding DA. Ultrastructure of a human nasal papilloma. Laryngoscope 1965;75:144–52.

[27] Ridolfi RL, Leiberman PH, Erlandson RA, et al. Schneiderian papillomas: a clinico–pathologic study of 30 cases. Am J Surg Pathol 1977;1:43–53.

[28] Costa J, Howley PM, Bowling MC, et al. Presence of human papilloma viral antigens in ju-venile multiple laryngeal papilloma. Am J Clin Pathol 1981;75:194–7.

[29] Strauss M, Jenson AB. Human papillomavirus in various lesions of the head and neck. Otolaryngol Head Neck Surg 1985;93:342–6.

[30] Respler DS, Jahn A, Pater A, et al. Isolation and characterization of papillomavirus DNA from nasal inverting (Schneiderian) papillomas. Ann Otol Rhinol Laryngol 1987;96:170–3.

[31] Weber RS, Shillitoe EJ, Robbins KT, et al. Prevalence of human papillomavirus in inverted nasal papillomas. Arch Otolaryngol Head Neck Surg 1988;114(1):23–6.

[32] Brandwein M, Steinberg B, Thung S, et al. Human papillomavirus 6/11 and 16/18 in Schnei-derian inverted papillomas. In situ hybridization with human papillomavirus RNA probes. Cancer 1989;63(9):1708–13.

[33] Skolnick EM, Loewy A, Friedman JE. Inverted papilloma of the nasal cavity. Arch Otolar-yngol 1966;84:83–9.

[34] Buchwald C, Nielsen LH, Nielsen PL, et al. Inverted papilloma: a follow-up study including primarily unacknowledged cases. Am J Otolaryngol 1989;10(4):273–81.

[35] Verner JL, Maguda TA, Yound JM. Epithelial papillomas of the nasal cavity and sinuses. Arch Otolaryngol 1959;70:574–8.

[36] Dolgin SR, Zaveri VD, Casiano RR, et al. Different opinions for treatment of inverting papilloma of the nose and paranasal sinuses: a report of 41 cases. Laryngoscope 1992;102: 231–6.

[37] Schlosser RJ, Mason JC, Gross CW. Aggressive endoscopic resection of inverted papilloma: an update. Otolaryngol Head Neck Surg 2001;125(1):49–53.

[38] Wolfe SG, Schlosser RJ, Bolger WE, et al. Endoscopic and endoscope-assisted resections of inverted sinonasal papillomas. Otolaryngol Head Neck Surg 2004;131(3):174–9.

[39] Han JK, Smith TL, Loehrl T, et al. An evolution in the management of sinonasal inverting papilloma. Laryngoscope 2001;111:1395–400.

[40] Lee JT, Bhuta S, Lufkin R, et al. Isolated inverting papilloma of the sphenoid sinus. Laryngoscope 2003;113:41–4.

[41] Som PM, Lawson W, Lidov MW. Simulated aggressive skull base erosion in response to be-nign sinonasal disease. Radiology 1991;180(3):755–9.

[42] Momose KJ, Weber AL, Goodman M, et al. Radiologic aspects of inverted papilloma. Radiology 1980;134:73–9.

[43] Pasquini E, Sciaretta V, Frank G, et al. Endoscopic treatment of benign tumors of the nose and paranasal sinuses. Otolaryngol Head Neck Surg 2004;131(3):180–6.

[44] Roobottom CA, Jewell FM, Kabala J. Primary and recurrent inverting papilloma: appear-ances with magnetic resonance imaging. Clin Radiol 1995;50(7):472–5.

[45] Yousem DM, Fellows DW, Kennedy DW, et al. Inverted papilloma: evaluation with MR imaging. Radiology 1992;185(2):501–5.

[46] Snyder RM, Perzin KH. Papillomatosis of nasal cavity and paranasal sinuses (inverted papilloma, squamous papilloma): a clinicopathologic study. Cancer 1972;30:668–90.

[47] Lasser A, Rothfeld PR, Shapiro RS. Epithelial papilloma and squamous cell carcinoma of the nasal cavity and paranasal sinuses: a clinicopathological study. Cancer 1976;38(6): 2503–10.

[48] Sukenik MA, Casiano R. Endoscopic medial maxillectomy for inverted papillomas of the paranasal sinuses: value of the intraoperative endoscopic examination. Laryngoscope 2000;110:39–42.

[49] Lawson W, Biller HF, Jacobson A, et al. The role of conservative surgery in the management of inverted papilloma. Laryngoscope 1983;93:148–55.

[50] Christensen WN, Smith RRL. Schneiderian papillomas: a clinicopathologic study of 67 cases. Hum Pathol 1986;17:393–9.

[51] Myers EN, Schramm VL, Barnes EL. Management of inverted papilloma of the nose and paranasal sinuses. Laryngoscope 1981;91:2071–84.

[52] Wormald PJ, Ooi E, van Hasselt A, et al. Endoscopic removal of sinonasal inverted papilloma including endoscopic medial maxillectomy. Laryngoscope 2003;113:867–73.

[53] Suh KW, Facer GW, Devine KD, et al. Inverting papilloma of the nose and paranasal sinuses. Laryngoscope 1977;87:35–46.

[54] Trible WM, Lekagui S. Inverting papilloma of the nose and paranasal sinuses: report of 30 cases. Laryngoscope 1971;81:663–8.

[55] Waitz G, Wigand M. Results of endoscopic sinus surgery for the treatment of inverted papillomas. Laryngoscope 1992;102:917–22.

[56] McCary WS, Gross CW, Reibel JF, et al. Preliminary report: endoscopic versus external surgery in the management of inverting papilloma. Laryngoscope 1994;104(4):415–9.

[57] Stankiewicz J, Girgis S. Endoscopic surgical treatment of nasal and paranasal sinus inverted papilloma. Otolaryngol Head Neck Surg 1993;109:989–95.

[58] Krouse JH. Development of a staging system for inverted papilloma. Laryngoscope 2000; 110:965–8.

[59] Sadeghi N, Al-Dhahri S, Manoukian JJ. Transnasal endoscopic medial maxillectomy for inverting papilloma. Laryngoscope 2003;113:749–53.

[60] Schlosser RJ, Zachmann G, Harrison S, et al. The endoscopic modified Lothrop: long-term follow-up on 44 patients. Am J Rhinol 2002;16(2):103–7.

ELSEVIER
SAUNDERS

Otolaryngol Clin N Am
39 (2006) 619–637

OTOLARYNGOLOGIC
CLINICS
OF NORTH AMERICA

Endoscopic Management
of Sinonasal Malignancy

Pete S. Batra, MD*, Martin J. Citardi, MD, FACS

Section of Nasal and Sinus Disorders, The Cleveland Clinic Head and Neck
Institute, 9500 Euclid Avenue, Cleveland, OH 44195

The advent of rigid telescopes has revolutionized the management of rhinologic disease. These instruments have been used as a diagnostic and therapeutic tool for paranasal sinus inflammatory disease since the 1970s [1–3]. Endoscopic techniques have been used for treating increasingly complex intranasal pathology, including nasolacrimal duct obstruction [4], cerebrospinal fluid (CSF) leaks/encephaloceles [5], dysthyroid orbitopathy [6], and optic neuropathy [7]. Recently endoscopic techniques have also been used successfully to manage selected tumors, including inverted papilloma [8], angiofibromas [9], and hypophyseal tumors [10].

The evolution of sophisticated surgical instrumentation and advances in computer-aided surgery (CAS) have facilitated the consideration of resection of sinonasal malignancy using minimally invasive endoscopic techniques. Endoscopic resection of sinonasal malignancy offers several important advantages over the open approaches, including unparalleled visualization that allows precise tumor removal. The endoscopic approach allows preservation of uninvolved structures, avoidance of facial incisions, and superior cosmesis.

This article reviews patient evaluation strategies, surgical techniques, and outcomes data for the minimally invasive endoscopic resection (MIER). MIER has emerged as an alternative to traditional craniofacial resection (tCFR). When endoscopic resection is combined with bifrontal craniotomy,

Dr. Batra is a consultant for Critical Therapeutics, Inc. (Lexington, MA) (2005–present). Dr. Citardi was a member of the scientific advisory board of CBYON (Mountain View, CA) during 1999–2003; he currently is a member of the scientific advisory board of GE Healthcare Navigation & Visualization (Lawrence, MA).

* Corresponding author.
E-mail address: batrap@ccf.org (P.S. Batra).

doi:10.1016/j.otc.2006.01.012
oto.theclinics.com

this procedure is best termed *endoscopic-assisted craniofacial resection* (EA-CFR).

Patient evaluation

History and physical examination

All patient evaluations commence with a detailed history and physical examination. Common presenting symptoms for sinonasal tumors include nasal airway obstruction, epistaxis, nasal discharge, headaches, and smell disturbances. More advanced tumors may extend into the orbit, resulting in blurry vision, diplopia, or proptosis. Extension into the skull base may result in neurologic dysfunction, including cranial neuropathies, as the tumors track along cranial nerves. The presenting symptoms can often be nonspecific and even suggestive of chronic rhinosinusitis; thus, a high index of suspicion is imperative for avoiding an inordinate delay in diagnosis.

Detailed head and neck examinations should be performed in all patients. Anterior rhinoscopy may show a nasal mass that occludes the nasal cavity. Extensive malignancies may present with bilateral nasal involvement. Oral cavity examination may show palatal erosion by maxillary sinus malignancy, and loose dentition may indicate involvement of the alveolar bone. Ocular examination should be performed to document visual acuity and extraocular muscle movement. Tumors with orbital invasion may present with ophthalmoplegia or proptosis. Cranial nerve examination is imperative to exclude neurologic involvement. Neck examination must be performed to determine regional lymphatic involvement.

Nasal endoscopy

Nasal endoscopy is an integral part of the physical examination. The rigid telescope offers the unique opportunity to use the same modality for diagnosis, tumor resection, and postoperative surveillance. In the office, endoscopy may show an exophytic, friable mass in the nasal cavity (Fig. 1). Examination should include evaluation of the nasopharynx to rule out contiguous involvement. Tumors may cause postobstructive sinusitis. Cultures can also be obtained through endoscopy and can serve as the basis for specific antibiotic therapy to minimize sinonasal inflammation and edema.

Office biopsy is often possible in cooperative patients who have accessible tumors. The surgeon should be prepared to control bleeding that may result from the biopsy. Monopolar or bipolar (preferably) cautery and packing materials should be available. Tumors of vascular origin or extensive lesions with orbital or skull base involvement are better suited for biopsy in the operating room.

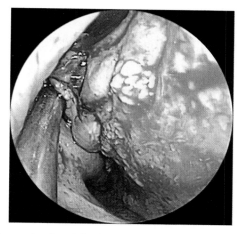

Fig. 1. Endoscopic image showing right sinonasal melanoma on the nasal septum. The right inferior turbinate also shows dark discoloration suggestive of melanoma.

Radiographic imaging

CT scans of the paranasal sinuses are performed in all patients. CT imaging is critical in defining the extent of the mass and its involvement of the contiguous structures. Often, CT shows a large soft-tissue mass that may fill the entire sinonasal cavity (Fig. 2). Bony erosion of the lamina papyracea and cribriform plate may be present, suggesting breach of the orbital or intracranial compartments, respectively (Fig. 3). The three-dimensional extent of the lesion and its involvement of the adjacent critical structures are defined by 1-mm axial cuts through the paranasal sinuses with coronal

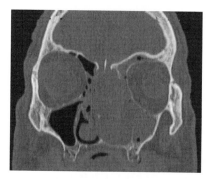

Fig. 2. Coronal sinus CT showing complete opacification of the left nasal cavity and adjacent sinuses. Because retained secretions and soft tissue have similar densities, the extent of the tumor cannot be discerned. Preoperative MRI and intraoperative findings confirmed that a large squamous cell carcinoma filled essentially all of the left ethmoid sinuses and nasal cavity, with displacement but not invasion of the nasal septum.

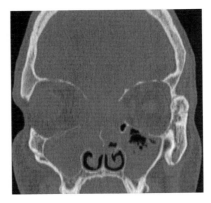

Fig. 3. Coronal sinus CT illustrating a large esthesioneuroblastoma with erosion of the medial orbital wall, the ethmoid roof, and the cribriform plate bilaterally. (The corresponding MR image is shown in Fig. 4.)

and sagittal reformatting. Preoperative triplanar review of the images at a computer workstation is imperative in formulating an effective surgical strategy for the patient.

MRI should be obtained in all patients who have extensive lesions. MRI, with its superior resolution of the soft-tissue structures, further defines the extent of the lesion. In cases of bony erosion of the orbit or skull base, MRI delineates the involvement of the orbital soft tissues and the dura, respectively (Fig. 4). MRI also differentiates actual paranasal sinus tumor involvement from postobstructive sinusitis.

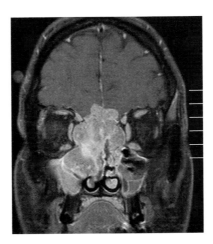

Fig. 4. Coronal MRI with contrast showing a large enhancing sinus mass. The tumor has violated the medial orbital walls, but seems to be pushing the orbital contents rather than invading them. Superiorly, the tumor seems to be at least focally invasive and probably overtly invasive of the dura and perhaps brain parenchyma. (The corresponding CT image is shown in Fig. 3.)

Positron emission tomography (PET) should be considered in all patients as part of the initial evaluation for metastatic disease. Distant metastatic disease may modify the management strategy from curative to palliative intent. In addition, preoperative PET imaging can serve as a baseline for comparison after surgical intervention, especially if unexpected areas of increased activity are noted [11]. Alternatively, a CT of the neck, chest, abdomen, and pelvis with contrast may be used to assess the presence of regional and distal metastases at presentation.

Surgical strategies and techniques for minimally invasive endoscopic resection

Multidisciplinary evaluation

Management of sinonasal malignancies is a multidisciplinary approach. The rhinologic sinus surgeon often plays a central role in facilitating patient care when the MIER approach is contemplated. Neurosurgery and ophthalmology should be recruited to address intracranial and orbital disease, respectively. The head and neck surgeon may be involved to address regional neck disease through neck dissection. Radiation and medical oncologists should be available for adjunctive radiotherapy and chemotherapy.

All cases should be discussed at a multidisciplinary tumor board if the treating institution sponsors such a meeting. The consensus that develops from the evaluations provided by the various specialists leads to a comprehensive treatment strategy for each patient. Patients should actively participate in this process so they understand the implications of sinonasal neoplasia and its treatment. If the MIER strategy is recommended, the rhinologic surgeon should explain that this is a relatively new paradigm that shows considerable promise. Of course, patients should have the option to undergo consultation to consider alternative approaches, including traditional "open" approaches.

In most instances, patients will undergo multimodality treatment postoperatively and even preoperatively. Thus, surgical intervention must be closely coordinated with medical and radiation oncology.

Oncologic strategy

The central principles of surgical oncology remain paramount in endoscopic resection of sinonasal malignancy. The goal of oncologic resection is complete tumor extirpation, which can be successfully achieved in many cases using the endoscopic technique. Next, the surgical goal must be achieved while minimizing adverse impact on patients' quality of life. For paranasal sinus malignancies, important functional considerations include preservation of neurologic function, vision, swallowing, voice, and a normal physical appearance. MIER may help attain the oncologic objectives with less functional morbidity than the open approaches [12].

When considering the MIER approach for tumor resection, a clear surgical plan must be devised. The objective should be successful tumor extirpation with acceptably low risk for complications. Thus, endoscopic and open approaches should be carefully considered for achieving this goal. The surgeon should be competent in both approaches. In this way, the surgeon can devise the best strategy to achieve the desired surgical objective. In particular, the surgeon should be able to incorporate traditional open approaches and newer endoscopic techniques into a specific procedure, if warranted.

Instrumentation

Appropriate surgical instrumentation is a requisite for endoscopic tumor resection. Because adequate visualization is critical, a three-chip endoscopic camera with digital enhancement, a high-quality, medical-grade monitor, and an assortment of 0°, 30°, 45°, and 70° telescopes should be available. Older video and endoscopic equipment, or equipment that has fallen into even mild levels of disrepair, will compromise visualization of subtle cues that guide complete resection. Furthermore, through-cutting instruments allow for bony cuts within the confines of the paranasal sinuses, and sharp, fine endoscopic scissors can be used for soft-tissue dissection, much as scissor dissection is an option for neck dissection.

Powered instrumentation, including soft-tissue shavers and surgical drills, facilitate rapid removal of soft-tissue and bone, respectively. Soft-tissue shaver tips are available in 40°, 60°, 90°, and 120° angles that facilitate tumor removal in maxillary and frontal sinuses. Using soft-tissue shavers in tumor resection fulfills two important purposes: 1) the constant suction helps clear blood and tumor cells, theoretically decreasing the risk for tumor seeding, and 2) the use of multiple traps serves to compartmentalize the tumor, thus creating a three-dimensional tumor map. The latest powered instrumentation supports drill rotation speeds of 12,000 rpm (or greater). Such speeds are critical for rapid but controlled removal of bone. The availability of diamond and cutting burrs at various angles is also important.

Bipolar cautery devices allow for hemostasis and minimize bloody contamination of the surgical field. Options for intranasal bipolar cautery include the Bi-Frazier Bipolar Suction cautery (Surgical Laser Technologies, Inc., Montgomeryville, Pennsylvania), the Landolt cautery (Aesculap Inc., Center Valley, Pennsylvania), and the Wormald Bipolar Forceps (Medtronic Xomed, Jacksonville, Florida). Use of monopolar cautery devices at the skull base and orbit should be discouraged because the heat and current transmission from monopolar cautery may easily damage adjacent structures.

Salvage of intraoperative blood loss and subsequent autotransfusion through Cell Saver technology (Haemonetics, Braintree, Massachusetts) should be considered. These devices collect hemorrhage, debris, and irrigation fluid from the operative field and then harvest the patient's own red blood cells for autotransfusion. The washing process before autotransfusion reduces the risk for transmission of infection and neoplastic cells to an acceptable level.

Computer-aided surgery

Over the past 15 years, CAS has been increasingly used in endoscopic sinus surgery [13,14]. CAS can be instrumental in facilitating precise endoscopic resection of sinonasal malignancy. Preoperative triplanar review of the images helps the surgeon understand the intimate relationship of the tumor to associated critical structures, including the orbit, cribriform plate, and pterygomaxillary or infratemporal fossa. Thus, the surgeon is able to formulate a more effective surgical plan and provide better preoperative patient counseling. Surgical navigation allows the preoperative imaging data and surgical plan to be directly correlated with the operative field, providing a better safety profile and thereby decreasing morbidity and increasing the efficacy of surgery.

Novel software applications further enhance the capabilities of the CAS technology. CT and MRI are essential for evaluation of sinonasal malignancy, especially in cases of skull base involvement. CT–MR fusion technology merges the two modalities to better delineate the extent of the tumor and its involvement of the contiguous paranasal sinus structures. This application can be used for preoperative planning and intraoperative surgical navigation for endoscopic approaches to the skull base (Figs. 5 and 6) [15].

Three-dimensional CT angiography offers an effective means for assessing the relationship of the skull base lesions to the internal carotid artery (ICA). The application of software filter and segmentation algorithms to the raw CT data provides unique ways for visualizing the skull base and vascular anatomy for diagnosis and preoperative assessment. Furthermore, these processed images may be incorporated into surgical navigation, thereby significantly improving the outcomes and reducing the morbidity of endoscopic skull base surgery when proximity to the ICA is a major surgical challenge (Fig. 7) [16].

Despite the tremendous technical advances in instrumentation and CAS, surgical expertise in advanced endoscopic techniques is the most important prerequisite when considering MIER.

Lumbar drainage

Perioperative use of a lumbar drain has engendered considerable controversy. Complications from lumbar drainage include meningitis and even cerebral herniation [17,18]. Some authors completely and routinely avoid lumbar drainage during anterior skull base surgery [19], whereas others use a drain preoperatively but remove it at the end of surgery [20]. Two strategies for lumbar drainage have emerged.

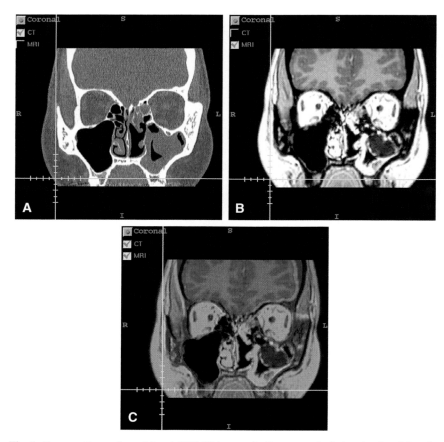

Fig. 5. Preoperative review of fused CT-MR images facilitates surgical planning by giving detailed information about tumor extension, as shown in this patient who has a low-grade malignant nerve sheath tumor of the left superior nasal cavity and posterior ethmoid. After three previous procedures, recurrent/persistent neoplasm is still present. (*A*) CT findings are nonspecific. (*B*) Tumor shows brighter signal intensity. (*C*) Fusion images show tumor as bright signal, and the integrity of the adjacent skull base is clear.

The first strategy advocates routine placement of a lumbar drain for all cases where a skull base defect is anticipated. After induction of general endotracheal anesthesia, the neurosurgery service places a lumbar drain in patients expected to undergo endoscopic cribriform plate and ethmoid roof resection or bifrontal craniotomy. This procedure permits decompression of the brain and facilitates management of intraoperative CSF leaks encountered during anterior skull base (ASB) resection.

The second strategy avoids routine placement of a lumbar drain. Instead, lumbar drainage is reserved only for special situations, including suspected elevated intracranial pressure, CSF leak in the immediate postoperative period, or problematic skull base reconstruction. At surgery, the

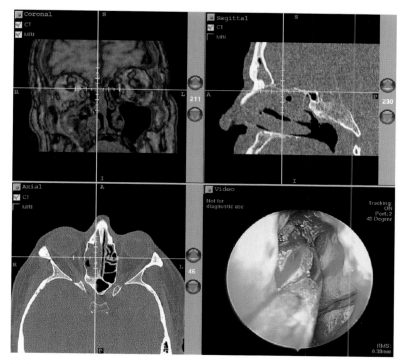

Fig. 6. CT-MR fusion images may be combined with surgical navigation. This still image capture was obtained during the computer-aided endoscopic resection of a right ethmoid adenocarcinoma. The upper left image is a fused CT-MR image, the lower right image is the standard endoscopic view, and the remaining quadrants show conventional CT images.

intraoperative leakage of CSF equalizes CSF pressure with ambient pressure; thus graft placement for reconstruction moves quickly after the flow of CSF through the skull base defect slows. The normalization of CSF pressures after graft placement is beneficial because re-expansion of the CSF-containing space holds the graft in position along the intracranial side of the defect. Details for skull base reconstruction are discussed later.

In the end, the decision for lumbar drainage occurs at the discretion of senior surgeon, who must consider various factors, including skull base defect characteristics (size and location) and potential drain morbidity.

Tracheostomy

In patients undergoing ASB resection, some surgeons recommend routine tracheostomy to divert airflow and decrease the risk for postoperative pneumocephalus. Practical experience has shown that the MIER approach without tracheotomy does not entail a greater risk for pneumocephalus.

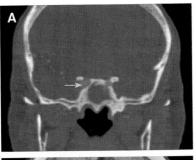

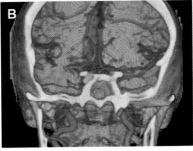

Fig. 7. Three-dimensional CT angiography provides information about the ICA at the skull base. (*A*) Contrast is seen in the right ICA. (*B*) The software has rendered a three-dimensional model of the ICA. This image has been rendered to show the bony skull anatomy and the contrast-filled ICA.

Specific operative techniques for tumor excision

MIER represents the integration of a wide variety of endoscopic procedures that have been developed since the introduction of surgical nasal endoscopy. In essence, MIER occurs when the surgeon selects the appropriate combination of endoscopic procedures to achieve complete tumor removal. Broadly, MIER encompasses two seemingly divergent surgical strategies. The first strategy may be termed the *outside-in approach*, in which the surgeon chooses to outflank the tumor by dissecting around the tumor, typically in a submucoperiosteal plane (Fig. 8). The second alternative is the *inside-out approach*, in which the core of large-bulky tumors is removed first and then the peripheral margins of the tumor are collapsed inward for removal (Fig. 9). In a few instances, the surgeon may choose only one of these strategies, but in most instances both strategies are used selectively in the same case.

Tumor removal for MIER requires the compulsive tracking of points of tumor attachment, which must be completely dissected to achieve sound surgical margins. The surgeon must develop a three-dimensional tumor map as the tumor is removed. Intraoperative frozen sections are frequently used to guide the resection; 20 or more frozen sections during MIER are not unusual.

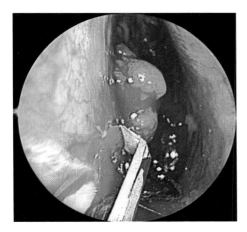

Fig. 8. Endoscopic image showing disposable round blade being used to make a mucosal cut on the right lateral nasal wall so that subperiosteal elevation of mucosa may commence. This "outside-in" approach is an important strategy for endoscopic resection of neoplasms.

Complete unilateral or, if clinically indicated, bilateral sphenoethmoidectomy and maxillary antrostomy are performed in most cases. Endoscopic septectomy may be required if the tumor involves the septum or to increase exposure within the paranasal sinus confines. Frontal sinusotomy or endoscopic frontal sinus drillout may be necessary to obtain the anterior margin for the tumor resection. Unilateral or bilateral endoscopic orbital decompression for removal of the orbital wall may be used to clear the lateral margins. Of course, direct extension into the orbit with invasion of the orbital

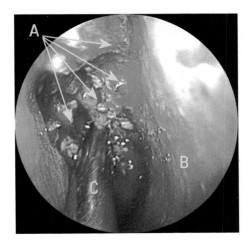

Fig. 9. Endoscopic image showing a bulky tumor (A) of the right nasal cavity (septum, [B]) being resected by removing its core with a microdebrider (C). This "inside-out" approach is an important strategy for endoscopic resection of neoplasms.

soft tissue contents may necessitate orbital exenteration. This procedure previously required open approaches, whereas more recently the minimally invasive approach using endoscopic power-assisted orbital exenteration has also been successful [21].

The skull base is usually addressed after the other parts of the tumor have been removed. Whether to resect the cribriform plate or ethmoid roof is generally decided intraoperatively. If the tumor extends to or frankly erodes this boundary, then resection of the cribriform plate or bony ethmoid roof is appropriate. Angled diamond burr tips can be instrumental in achieving precise and atraumatic resection of this bony margin. Cutting burrs should be avoided on the skull base because they may cause inadvertent tearing of the dura and even intracranial injury. After bone removal, the dural may be sampled for frozen section. If the frozen section shows neoplasm, then dural resection is required. If the tumor has no evidence of extensive transdural violation, endoscopic dural resection should be considered (Fig. 10); however, intraoperative consultation with neurosurgery should be obtained. Extensive dural or direct intraparenchymal involvement cannot be cleared strictly through the MIER technique. In these cases, bifrontal craniotomy is required for clearing the superior margin of the tumor.

Skull base reconstruction

CSF leaks are expected sequelae for cribriform plate resection, and CSF leaks are common after removal of the ethmoid roof. All CSF leaks should

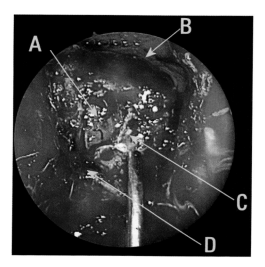

Fig. 10. Endoscopic image showing resection of the dura overlying the ethmoid roof and cribriform plate. (*A*) Exposed brain. (*B*) Frontal sinus. (*C*) Incised dural flap before its removal. (*D*) Cut anterior ethmoid artery.

be identified and repaired intraoperatively to avoid any adverse long-term effects. Layered reconstruction of the anterior skull base is the most effective technique, and a three-layered reconstruction is the preferred technique [22]. The dura should be carefully elevated circumferentially to allow for placement of autogenous fascia or acellular dermal allograft (Alloderm, LifeCell Corporation, The Woodlands, Texas), which is placed as an underlay graft. Septal/conchal cartilage/bone or split calvarial bone graft may be used to support the skull base to prevent iatrogenic encephalocele formation. Free bone grafts have been associated with extrusion after radiation therapy, and therefore the surgeon may choose to omit this layer in selected cases. A second layer of fascia or acellular dermal allograft should be placed in a similar fashion (Fig. 11). Free mucosal grafts from the septum or floor of nose should be used as an overlay graft to complete the layered reconstruction. Fibrin glue or a similar surgical sealant (Tisseel, Baxter Health care Corporation, Deerfield, Illinois) can hold the mucosal graft in place. The entire reconstruction should be supported with nasal packing, including FloSeal (Baxter Health care Corporation, Deerfield, Illinois), Gelfoam (Johnson & Johnson, Somerville, New Jersey), Surgiflo (Johnson & Johnson, Somerville, New Jersey), and expandable nasal tampon sponges (Merocel, Medtronic Xomed, Jacksonville, Florida). Of course, the surgeon must harvest any autogenous grafts from intranasal sites far from the neoplasm to avoid inadvertent seeding of the reconstruction with tumor cells.

If a bifrontal craniotomy is performed, the reconstruction is different. In most instances, a pericranial flap will suffice for closure; however, in a previously irradiated field, a vascularized free flap should be considered strongly.

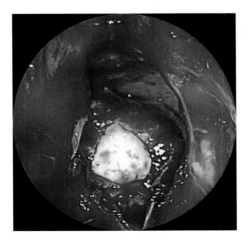

Fig. 11. After dural resection, skull base reconstruction should entail placement of multiple layers of graft material. This endoscopic image shows the second layer of acellular dermal allograft used for closure of the defect shown in Fig. 10.

Postoperative care

Most patients undergoing the MIER approach without skull base resection are observed overnight and can be discharged the following day. If the dura has been exposed or lumbar drain has been placed, patients are transferred to the neurosurgical floor for drain care and monitoring. A postoperative head CT should be obtained at the discretion of the senior surgeon. Indications for this imaging study include significant dural bleeding and a difficult skull base reconstruction. If a lumbar drain has been placed, it is maintained for 3 to 5 days. Intravenous antibiotics (first-generation cephalosporin or vancomycin) are continued while the lumbar drain is in place. Long-term prophylactic antibiotics are discouraged because of concerns about inducing antimicrobial resistance. Prophylactic antibiotics with meningeal penetration are not routinely used unless the operative field was significantly infected and bacterial seeding of the intracranial space is a concern.

Nonabsorbable nasal packing is left in place for 3 to 5 days and generally removed in the office. Meticulous sinonasal debridement is initiated 1 week after surgery. However, the skull base reconstruction is not manipulated for weeks to allow for complete healing. Any postoperative bacterial sinusitis episodes are treated aggressively with culture-directed antibiotics (oral and topical). In most instances, intranasal crusting persists for at least several weeks after surgery, but this crusting generally improves gradually because it is débrided under endoscopic visualization and as the patient performs gentle nasal irrigations with saline. Adjunctive treatment, such as radio- or chemotherapy, is also started approximately 3 to 4 weeks after surgery.

Long-term monitoring of these patients is essential. Such monitoring includes serial nasal endoscopy for the primary site. In addition, repeat imaging studies should also be preformed. In general, a repeat brain/orbit/sinus MR scan with and without intravenous contrast should be obtained 3 to 4 months after completion of all therapy, including radiation therapy and chemotherapy (Fig. 12). Repeat metastatic workup, including body CT and PET scans, may be obtained at the same time. This battery of imaging studies should be performed again at 6-month intervals for approximately 2 years and then regularly thereafter at the discretion of the senior surgeon. Because recurrent neoplasms at the primary site are difficult to distinguish from anticipated postoperative changes and changes caused by radiotherapy and chemotherapy, comparisons among imaging studies obtained over time are necessary to exclude recurrent tumor.

Outcomes

Published reports for endoscopic management of sinonasal malignancy have increased over the past few years. Initial studies from Europe have reported promising results. Goffart and colleagues [23] reported on 78 patients

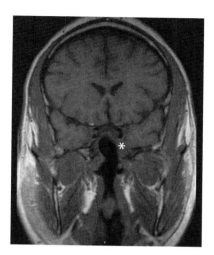

Fig. 12. Coronal MR obtained 20 months after endoscopic resection and postoperative radiation therapy for left sphenoid adenoid cystic carcinoma shows changes that may be equivocal for recurrent tumor with thickening of the left cavernous sinus (indicated by *). Because the previous MR scans have shown no progression of this abnormality and the endoscopic examination is unremarkable, this patient is considered to be "tumor-free." Nonetheless, close regular follow-up is planned.

who had sinonasal malignancies, with adenocarcinoma the most common histopathology. In this series, 66 patients underwent an exclusive endoscopic resection, whereas 9 patients needed to undergo a craniotomy and another 3 patients a limited orbital resection. Overall survival was 73.1% and 54.9% and disease-free survival was 54.9% and 52.3% at 2 and 5 years, respectively. Additionally, the researchers noted that the adenocarcinoma group showed a significantly better prognosis than other histologic types, with 2- and 5-year survival rates of 89.8% and 63.8%, respectively.

Stammberger and colleagues [24] reported on 36 patients treated with a strictly transnasal endoscopic approach. This study includes patients who had a diverse range of malignant neoplasms, but esthesioneuroblastoma was the most common tumor (n = 8). The authors noted that the outcomes were similar to the open approaches. Additionally, 100% disease-free survival was reported for all 8 patients who had esthesioneuroblastoma treated with combined endoscopic resection and gamma knife radiosurgery. In a more recent update, these authors report 100% survival at a median follow-up of 58 months for 14 patients who had esthesioneuroblastoma treated with endoscopic resection and postoperative gamma knife radiotherapy [25].

Roh and colleagues [26] published the first substantial experience with the endoscopic techniques for sinonasal malignancy in the United States. These authors describe 19 patients who had sinonasal malignancy treated using endoscopic techniques. Thirteen patients were treated exclusively with the endoscopic approach (MIER), whereas 6 patients were treated in conjunction with neurosurgery (EA-CFR). Combined radiation with or without chemotherapy was used in 15 of 19 (78.9%) cases. The local recurrence and distant metastasis rates were 26.3% and 15.8%, respectively. Overall survival rate was 78.9% at 32.1 months and disease-free survival rate by clinical, endoscopic, and radiographic surveillance was 68.4% at 33.1 months.

Scattered case reports and case series have attested to the feasibility of the endoscopic approach for ASB malignancy [27–30]. The initial study by Yuen and colleagues [27] reported a 1-year disease-free survival after resection of a persistent esthesioneuroblastoma after radiation therapy using the endoscopic approach. Other researchers have also reported on the efficacy of the endoscopic approach for esthesioneuroblastomas. Unger and colleagues [28] reported on 6 patients who had esthesioneuroblastomas treated with endoscopic skull base resection followed by gamma knife radiosurgery. Tumor control was achieved in all patients who had median follow-up of 57 months. Similarly, Casiano and colleagues [29] reported on 5 patients who had Kadish stage A or B esthesioneuroblastomas. All patients underwent endoscopic ASB resection with no local recurrences, although 2 patients developed regional metastasis (orbit and neck). Overall, an 80% disease-free survival was reported at 31 months.

Most recently, Batra and colleagues [12] compared MIER with tCFR for treatment of ASB neoplasms. In this study, 9 patients underwent management with MIER and 16 with tCFR. The researchers observed no statistical differences between the groups in operative time, blood loss, and hospital stay, whereas they observed major complications in 22% and 44% of the patients in the MIER and CFR groups, respectively. Recurrence was noted in 33% and 36% of patients in the MIER and CFR groups, respectively. Mortality rates in the MIER and CFR subsets were 0% and 27%, respectively. This collective experience suggests that MIER of sinonasal malignancy may be a viable alternative to traditional open approaches.

Discussion

The MIER technique has several advantages that make it an attractive alternative to open approaches for managing sinonasal malignancy. The superb visualization and magnification afforded by the rigid telescopes offer significant advantages. The nasal telescopes facilitate the unique opportunity for precise tumor removal and preservation of uninvolved structures (thus avoiding the so-called "collateral damage" intrinsic to the open approaches). Endoscopic visualization allows unparalleled views of the sphenoid and orbital apex, making lesions in this area more readily amenable to resection. Tumor margins can be determined with greater confidence, especially at the sinonasal–orbital interface when considering orbital exenteration, and at the sinonasal–dural margin when considering tCFR or EA-CFR. The avoidance of facial incisions allows for superior cosmesis, which may be an important consideration for some patients.

The limitations of MIER must also be appropriately considered. Technical requisites and endoscopic expertise are absolute requirements for MIER. The only absolute contraindication to the endoscopic approach is invasion of the facial soft tissues with malignancy; these patients are better served with open approaches (if surgical resection is even warranted). Relative contraindications to the MIER technique include massive bilateral disease, highly vascular tumors, need for orbital exenteration, and lateral tumor extension into the pterygomaxillary space or infratemporal fossa. These clinical scenarios require even greater endoscopic expertise and may be successfully managed by experienced endoscopic surgeons. Until further experience is gained, utmost caution must be exercised when considering MIER in this subset of patients. Of course, if an open approach is warranted, the surgeon may still include some endoscopic techniques if portions of the procedure are amenable to endoscopic resection.

Perhaps the biggest concern in using the endoscopic approach is the difficulty in performing an en bloc resection. Theoretically, a piecemeal resection could result in intraoperative tumor seeding and increase the risk for local recurrence; however, this concern has not been realized in practice. The aforementioned studies have reported recurrence and disease-free survival rates that are comparable with open approaches. Furthermore, the likelihood of en bloc resection by the traditional CFR has been questioned. McCutcheon and colleagues [31] have reported that "...as the tumor is usually removed in a piecemeal fashion, the chances for residual microscopic disease are significant...Given the anatomic limitations of this region, however, the oncologic ideal of a wide, en bloc resection was rarely achieved...." Thus, the open CFR approach with piecemeal resection did not seem to compromise survival in their patients who had ASB malignancy. The fundamental limitation for en bloc resection reflects two features of these neoplasms: 1) their location prohibits wide margins, which would potentially sacrifice many uninvolved but critical normal structures (eg, brain, orbit, cranial nerves), and 2) the ethmoid bone where most of the lesions originate is intrinsically flimsy and the neoplasm further destroys this structure; thus, holding the specimen in one piece during resection is inherently challenging.

Summary

Advancements in endoscopic visualization and instrumentation have facilitated the application of endoscopic techniques for the resection of anterior skull base neoplasms. Initial experiences with the endoscopic excision of benign neoplasms suggested that more aggressive malignant neoplasms are also amenable to endoscopic resection. Early anecdotal reports and larger retrospective series have confirmed that endoscopic resection of malignant neoplasms is feasible and offers oncologic results similar to traditional open approaches. The endoscopic strategy requires specific equipment and an experienced rhinologic surgeon, and all patients should undergo a comprehensive, multidisciplinary evaluation. Therefore, for selected patients who have sino-nasal malignancy, endoscopic resection should be considered a viable alternative that offers adequate surgical access, good clinical outcomes, and reduced patient morbidity.

References

[1] Kennedy D. Functional endoscopic sinus surgery. Technique. Arch Otolaryngol 1985; 111(10):643–9.

[2] Stammberger H. Endoscopic endonasal surgery–concepts in treatment of recurring rhinosinusitis. Part II. Surgical technique. Otolaryngol Head Neck Surg 1986;94(2):147–56.

[3] Wigand ME. Transnasal ethmoidectomy under endoscopical control. Rhinology 1981;19(1): 7–15.

[4] Metson R. Endoscopic surgery for lacrimal obstruction. Otolaryngol Head Neck Surg 1991; 104(4):473–9.

[5] Lanza DC, O'Brien DA, Kennedy DW. Endoscopic repair of cerebrospinal fluid fistulae and encephaloceles. Laryngoscope 1996;106(9 Pt 1):1119–25.

[6] Kennedy DW, Goodstein ML, Miller NR, et al. Endoscopic transnasal orbital decompression. Arch Otolaryngol Head Neck Surg 1990;116(3):275–82.

[7] Luxenberger W, Stammberger H, Jebeles JA, et al. Endoscopic optic nerve decompression: the Graz experience. Laryngoscope 1998;108(6):873–82.

[8] Tufano RP, Thaler ER, Lanza DC, et al. Endoscopic management of sinonasal inverted papilloma. Am J Rhinol 1999;13(6):423–6.

[9] Carrau RL, Snyderman CH, Kassam AB, et al. Endoscopic and endoscopic-assisted surgery for juvenile angiofibroma. Laryngoscope 2001;111(3):483–7.

[10] Nasseri SS, Kasperbauer JL, Strome SE, et al. Endoscopic transnasal pituitary surgery: report on 180 cases. Am J Rhinol 2001;15(4):281–7.

[11] McGuirt WF, Greven K, Williams D III, et al. PET scanning in head and neck oncology: a review. Head Neck 1998;20(3):208–15.

[12] Batra PS, Citardi MJ, Worley S, et al. Resection of anterior skull base tumors: comparison of combined traditional and endoscopic techniques. Am J Rhinol 2005;19(5):521–8.

[13] Olson G, Citardi MJ. Image-guided functional endoscopic sinus surgery. Otolaryngol Head Neck Surg 2000;123(3):188–94.

[14] Citardi MJ, Batra PS. Image-guided sinus surgery: current concepts and technology. Otolaryngol Clin North Am 2005;38(3):439–52.

[15] Leong JL, Batra PS, Citardi MJ. CT-MR fusion for the management of skull base lesions. Otolaryngol Head Neck Surg, in press.

[16] Leong JL, Batra PS, Citardi MJ. Three-dimensional computed tomography angiography of the internal carotid artery for preoperative evaluation of sinonasal lesions and intraoperative surgical navigation. Laryngoscope 2005;115(9):1618–23.

[17] Roland PS, Marple BF, Meyerhoff WL, et al. Complications of lumbar spinal fluid drainage. Otolaryngol Head Neck Surgery 1992;107:564–9.

[18] Francel PC, Persing JA, Cantrell RW, et al. Neurological deterioration after lumbar cerebrospinal fluid drainage. J Carniofac Surg 1992;3:145–8.

[19] Har-El G, Casiano RR. Endoscopic management of anterior skull base tumors. Otolaryngol Clin North Am 2005;38:133–44.

[20] Kraus DH, Shah JP, Arbit E, et al. Complications of craniofacial resection for tumors involving the anterior skull base. Head Neck 1995;16:307–12.

[21] Batra PS, Lanza DC. Endoscopic power-assisted orbital exenteration. Am J Rhinol 2005; 19(3):297–301.

[22] Lorenz RR, Dean RL, Hurley DB, et al. Endoscopic reconstruction of anterior and middle cranial fossa defects using acellular dermal allograft. Laryngoscope 2003;113(3):496–501.

[23] Goffart Y, Jorissen M, Daele J, et al. Minimally invasive endoscopic management of malignant sinonasal tumours. Acta Otorhinolaryngol Belg 2000;54(2):221–32.

[24] Stammberger H, Anderhuber W, Walch C, et al. Possibilities and limitations of endoscopic management of nasal and paranasal sinus malignancies. Acta Otorhinolaryngol Belg 1999; 53(3):199–205.

[25] Unger F, Haselsberger K, Walch C, et al. Combined endoscopic surgery and radiosurgery as treatment modality for olfactory neuroblastoma (esthesioneuroblastoma). Acta Neurochir (Wien) 2005;147:595–602.

[26] Roh HJ, Batra PS, Citardi MJ, et al. Endoscopic resection of sinonasal malignancies: a preliminary report. Am J Rhinol 2004;18(4):239–46.

[27] Yuen AP, Fung CF, Hung KN. Endoscopic cranionasal resection of anterior skull base tumors. Am J Otolaryngol 1997;18(6):431–3.

[28] Unger F, Walch C, Stammberger H, et al. Olfactory neuroblastoma (esthesioneuroblastoma): report of six cases treated by a novel combination of endoscopic surgery and radiosurgery. Minim Invasive Neurosurg 2001;44(2):79–84.

[29] Casiano RR, Numa WA, Falquez AM. Endoscopic resection of esthesioneuroblastoma. Am J Rhinol 2001;15(4):271–9.

[30] Kuhn FA, Javer AR. Low-grade fibrosarcoma of the anterior skull base: endoscopic resection and repair. Am J Rhinol 2003;17(6):347–50.

[31] McCutcheon IE, Blacklock JB, Weber RS, et al. Anterior transcranial (craniofacial) resection of tumors of the paranasal sinuses: surgical technique and results. Neurosurgery 1996;38(3):471–9.

OTOLARYNGOLOGIC
CLINICS
OF NORTH AMERICA

Otolaryngol Clin N Am
39 (2006) 639–656

Transnasal Endoscopic Surgical Approaches to the Clivus

Aldo Cassol Stamm, MD[a,b,*],
Shirley S.N. Pignatari, MD[a,b], Eduardo Vellutini, MD[c]

[a]*Federal University of São Paulo, Paulista School of Medicine, São Paulo, Brazil*
[b]*São Paulo ENT Center, Hospital Professor Edmundo Vasconcelos, Rua Afonso Braz 525
CJ13, São Paulo, Brazil 04511-010*
[c]*Department of Neurosurgery, Hospital Oswaldo Cruz, São Paulo, Brazil*

Management of lesions involving the clival region has changed dramatically since the introduction of transnasal microscopic and endoscopic techniques using new advanced surgical instrumentation. However, effective and safe treatment of lesions involving the skull base is still challenging [1]. Several approaches using microscopic surgical techniques have been proposed, seeking to optimize the exposure and minimize the risk of complications. All such microscopic anterior skull base approaches aim to avoid nerve and brain retraction and have been developed along two basic anterior midline routes: the transoral and the transnasal [2,3,4]. The current goal of surgical approaches is to be straighter and faster, avoiding extensive cerebral retraction and presenting a lower rate of morbidity compared with that of classic approaches [5,6].

Nevertheless, despite lower morbidity and fewer complications, the problems of infection, cerebrospinal fluid (CSF) leakage, difficulty controlling intradural bleeding, and lack of appropriate surgical instruments still exist. One of the most difficult remaining challenges is the repair of large dural defects [1].

Surgical anatomy

Any transnasal endoscopic surgical approach to the clival region will necessarily involve the sphenoid sinus, and therefore anatomic knowledge of this paranasal sinus is imperative.

* Corresponding author.
E-mail address: centrodeorl@osite.com.br (A.C. Stamm).

Sphenoid sinus

The sphenoid sinus varies in shape and size and is asymmetrically divided into two parts by an irregular septum. The thin lateral wall of the well-developed sphenoid sinus forms the medial wall of the cavernous sinus. The intracavernous portion of the internal carotid artery (ICA) is the most medial structure within the cavernous sinus and, in well-developed sphenoid sinuses, produces a bony elevation in the lateral wall of the sinus called the carotid prominence. The carotid prominence is divided into presellar, infrasellar, and retrosellar segments [7]. The presellar segment corresponds with the anterior vertical segment and the anterior bend of the intracavernous portion of the ICA. The infrasellar segment corresponds with the short horizontal portion of the carotid, and the retrosellar segment reflects the posterior bend and posterior vertical segment.

The optic canal is often partially encircled by the sphenoid sinus and creates a bony bulge in the superoanterior portion of its lateral wall. The bony depression between the optic canal and the presellar segment of the carotid prominence is called the *opticocarotid recess* and extends a variable distance into the optic strut. The bony lateral sphenoid sinus wall over the ICA and the optic nerve is usually very thin and may be absent in some areas. Although Lang [8] observed that the canal of the optic nerve was dehiscent in 6% of cases, Seibert [9] found that the canal of the optic nerve bulged into the sphenoid sinus in 57% of cases and that 1% had no bony canal. Seibert [9] also noted that the horizontal portion of the intracavernous carotid artery extended prominently into the sphenoid sinus in 67% of cases and its bony covering was dehiscent in 6%. In his series, the maxillary nerve was prominent in the sphenoid sinus in 48% of specimens and dehiscent in 5%, and the pterygoid nerve (vidian) was prominent 18% of the time.

Clivus

The clivus separates the nasopharynx from the posterior cranial fossa. It is composed of the posterior portion of the sphenoid body (basisphenoid) and the basilar part of the occipital bone (basiocciput) and is further subdivided into upper, middle, and lower thirds. The upper third of the clivus is at the level of the sphenoid sinus and is formed by the basisphenoid bone, including the dorsum sella. The middle clivus corresponds with the rostral part of the basiocciput and is located above a line connecting the caudal ends of the petroclival fissures. The lower third of the clivus is formed by the caudal part of the basiocciput. The intracranial surface of the upper two thirds of the clivus faces the pons and is concave from side to side.

The extracranial surface of the clivus gives rise to the pharyngeal tubercle at the junction of the middle and lower clivus. The upper clivus faces the roof of the nasopharynx that extends downward in the midline to the level of the pharyngeal tubercle (Fig. 1A, B).

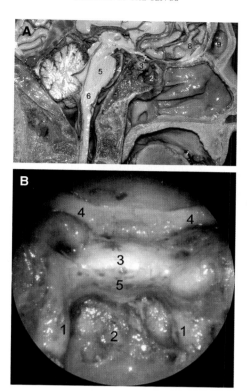

Fig. 1. (A) Midline sagittal section of the nasal cavity, sphenoid sinus, clivus, and adjacent structures (1, clivus; 2, sphenoid sinus; 3, pituitary gland; 4, basilar artery; 5, pons; 6, medulla; 7, optic nerve; 8, frontal lobe; 9, frontal sinus). (B) Endoscopic view of the posterior wall of the sphenoid sinus (1, prominence of the internal carotid arteries; 2, clivus; 3, anterior sellar wall; 4, optic nerves; 5, intercavernous sinus).

The upper and middle clivus are separated from the petrous portion of the temporal bone on each side by the petroclival fissure. The basilar venous plexus is situated between the two layers of the dura of the upper clivus and is related to the dorsum sella and the posterior wall of the sphenoid sinus. It forms interconnecting venous channels among the inferior petrosal sinuses laterally, the cavernous sinuses superiorly, and the marginal sinus and epidural venous plexus inferiorly. The basilar sinus is the largest communicating channel between the paired cavernous sinuses.

The average distance between the left and right internal carotid arteries just below the tuberculum sellae where they are closest to each other is 13.9 mm (range, 10–17 mm). At the anterior wall of the sella, the carotid arteries are separated by a distance of 20 mm (range, 13–26.5 mm) and by that of 17.4 mm (range, 10.5–26.5 mm) at the level of the clivus [7]. Jho and Ha [10] found the average width between the carotid arteries at the sellar floor level to be 16 mm (range 12–22 mm), and 19 mm (range 14–23 mm) at the lower end of the carotid arteries.

Retroclival region

Although most of the structures of the suprasellar area, cavernous sinus, and retrosphenoid sinus can be reached through the sphenoid sinus, the transnasal transclival endoscopic anatomy of the basal cisterns and posterior fossa through this sinus are not familiar to many surgeons [11].

When all the bone of the posterior and lateral walls of the sphenoid sinus has been removed, only periosteum covers the underlying anatomy. The tectorial membrane protects the clival dura in the middle and lower clivus. When the external layer of the dura is opened, the basilar venous plexus and cranial nerve VI on each side can be seen. The average distance between the abducens nerves (cranial nerve VI) at the dural emergence is 19.8 mm [12].

After opening the inner layer of the clival dura, the 0° endoscope shows the vertebral arteries, basilar artery and its branches (superior cerebellar arteries, anterior inferior cerebellar arteries [AICA]), posterior cerebral arteries, brain stem, mammillary bodies, and intradural pathway of cranial nerves III, IV, V, and VI. Just above the pituitary gland, the pituitary stalk, optic nerves, and optic chiasm can be seen. By introducing a 30°- or 45°-angled endoscope, the cerebellopontine angle, cranial nerves VII and VIII, lower cranial nerves, and retrosellar region (Fig. 2) can be viewed.

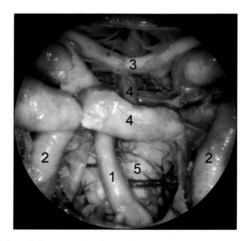

Fig. 2. Endoscopic view of the posterior fossa after the removal of the posterior wall of sphenoid sinus and upper clivus (1, basilar artery; 2, internal carotid arteries; 3, optic nerves and chiasm; 4, pituitary gland and pituitary stalk; 5, brainstem).

Preoperative evaluation

The success of any skull base procedure depends on several factors, including a thorough clinical history, a careful preoperative evaluation, a well-developed surgical plan, and physician–patient conversations that include a frank discussion of the diagnosis, surgical plan, possible complications, and physician and patient roles in the anticipated postoperative care plan.

Physical examination includes endoscopic assessment of the nasal cavity performed with the patient in a semisitting position. The nasal cavity is prepared with a topical anesthetic solution containing a vasoconstrictor. The examination is performed with rigid 4-mm 0° and 45° endoscopes. The flexible 3.2-mm endoscope is preferable for children and a straight 2.7-mm endoscope is occasionally used.

Preoperative image studies should include coronal, axial, and sagittal CT images of the sinuses and skull base as essential parts of the assessment of all skull base lesions. In addition to diagnostic information, CT permits assessment of critical anatomic information important during surgery, such as the presence and extent of erosions of the skull base; integrity of the medial orbital wall; position of the anterior skull base vessels; integrity and degree of aeration of the paranasal sinuses (particularly the sphenoid sinus); location and presence of intersinus septae; position of the internal carotid arteries, optic nerves, and cavernous sinuses; relationships among the ethmoid sinuses and the orbits and optic nerves; relationship between the roof of the ethmoid sinuses and the cribriform plate; and the presence of an Onodi cell. When used in conjunction with an image guidance system, the CT can also provide three-dimensional reconstruction of the patient's skull base region during surgery.

MRI is important in showing the morphology of the soft tissues and the presence of fluid, but is not helpful in assessing bony architecture. MRI helps differentiate between neoplastic or inflammatory tissue and retained secretions, and clarify the diagnosis of skull base malformations when meningoencephalocele, meningocele, or nasal gliomas are suspected. MRI is also valuable in patients who have erosion of the lateral sphenoid wall.

Magnetic resonance angiography (MRA) assesses the structure of medium to large arteries and should be considered for visualizing the relationship between the basilar and internal carotid arteries in patients who have erosion of the lateral and posterior sphenoid walls.

Angio-CT is a recent technology that allows simultaneous visualization of bony and vascular structures. Venous and arterial structures can be seen separately (venous phase and arterial phase) or together (part venous phase and part arterial phase). Angio-CT is especially useful in assessing the internal carotid and vertebrobasilar systems. Venous structures of particular surgical interest include the cavernous sinus, inferior and superior intercavernous sinuses, and the basilar venous plexus. This technology allows

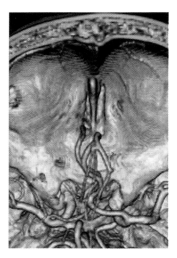

Fig. 3. Three-dimensional model of an angio CT showing anterior cranium seen from above and showing the relationships between the internal carotid and the vertebrobasilar arterial systems.

surgeons to better plan any surgical procedure, especially those involving the parasphenoidal regions and the anterior skull base (Fig. 3).

Although conventional angiography is not routinely performed, it can provide essential information in some specific situations. If a lesion is suspected to involve, impinge on, or displace the ICA, the surgeon must have accurate preoperative knowledge of the position of the ICA and its relationship to the lesion, especially when the transnasal transsphenoidal approach is contemplated (ie, accessing the skull base through the posterior and lateral wall of the sphenoid sinus). Angiography is also helpful for verifying the functional integrity of the circle of Willis, determining the extent of any carotid artery narrowing or occlusion, and differentiating an aneurysm from a tumor.

Operative technique

The patient is prepared as usual for transnasal endoscopic-assisted surgery. The patient is positioned supine on the operating table with the dorsum elevated 30° and the head extended 15° and turned toward the surgeon. No head fixation is necessary.

Transnasal endoscopic-assisted surgery of the skull base is performed under general controlled hypotensive anesthesia. Cottonoids containing adrenaline 1:2000 are placed in the nasal cavity, especially over the areas of surgical access. These cottonoids are left in place for approximately 10 minutes before the surgical procedure begins. If the surgical access is through the nasal septum, the septum is infiltrated with lidocaine with adrenaline 1:100.000. If necessary, adrenaline-soaked cottonoids are used for hemostasis during the surgery. If a CSF fistula is suspected, intrathecal fluorescein can be introduced at the beginning of the surgical procedure to facilitate its precise location [13]. If an image-guided system may be used, the headframe is set up for calibration.

Instrumentation

Clivus surgical procedures are performed with the endoscopes attached to an endocamera and a video monitor system. Most commonly, 4-mm endoscopes of 0° and 45° are used. In conjunction with Karl Storz Inc., we are developing a 5-mm wide-angled 0° telescope for these procedures to increase the field of view and illumination. Although conventional surgical instrumentation can also be used, most of the microendoscopic surgical instruments for these cases are slightly longer and thinner, but just as strong or stronger. Most have an articulation located at the edge, allowing adequate visualization of the operative field. Extra-long handpieces for the surgical drill are essential and are used almost exclusively with diamond burrs of various sizes. Medtronic Xomed has developed a new generation of high-speed drills that incorporate suction–irrigation functions to reduce operative time and allow more accurate dissection. Our initial experience has been very promising. Suction cannulas should have a blunted edge to avoid unnecessary trauma and mucosal bleeding. Contemporary suction elevators for septoplasty can elevate and cut tissue, aspirate blood, and allow the surgeon to operate the suction elevator with one hand while holding the endoscope with the other. Initial evaluation of the structures can be accomplished with a double-ended probe called a *seeker/palpator*. A Freer elevator is another useful instrument that has semisharp and blunt ends. The semisharp end can incise and dissect the mucosa, whereas the blunt end can be used to palpate and displace structures of the nasal cavity, such as the middle turbinate.

Monopolar and bipolar electrocautery permit the surgeon to control bleeding during the surgical access (bleeding from the incision of the nasal septum and from the septal artery that lies on the anterior wall of sphenoid sinus). Bleeding from the basilar venous plexus is not coagulated. Compression with Surgicel packing (Johnson & Johnson, New Brunswick, New Jersey) and obliteration of involved bony channels using diamond burrs or bone wax are helpful. Only a bipolar system of coagulation should be used to control venous or arterial intradural bleeding.

Powered instrumentation (eg, microdebriders) was initially developed for soft-tissue shaving and represents a major advance in transnasal endoscopic-assisted surgery. The instruments have multiple functions, including suction, cutting, and irrigation. Newer instruments with curved blades and burrs are able to remove bone and debulk some tumors. The newer microdebriders also produce a more precise cut of the diseased tissue, avoiding mucosal stripping, and are accompanied by continuous irrigation that improves visualization and diminishes blood loss. The new image guidance systems are precise and have been very helpful in some cases of clivus surgery. These systems of tridimensional navigation provide important information about the location of anatomic structures in the operative field and create an individual anatomic map generated from a preoperative CT. They are particularly useful in identifying the ICA and in accessing the petrous apex when lesions such as cholesterol granuloma are present. This system reduces the chances of surgical complications because it provides the surgeon with an exact anatomic location of a surgical instrument [1,14].

Transnasal–transsphenoidal surgical approaches to the clivus

Several transnasal–transsphenoidal approaches to the clivus have been described [15], including the transnasal direct and transseptal (combined with or without a transethmoidal approach). The choice of the appropriate transnasal technique for each patient depends on the nature, location, and extent of the lesion.

The clival bone can be removed from the floor of the sella to the foramen magnum in the craniocaudal dimension and laterally from one to another ICA with a high-speed drill. When the distance between the two internal carotid arteries is narrow, the transclival surgical access to the posterior fossa is much more difficult.

We use the following classification for transnasal surgical approaches:

1. Transnasal direct
2. Transseptal (anterior incision, posterior incision)
3. Transnasal with removal of the posterior part of the nasal septum (two-nostril approach).
4. Transnasal combined with transethmoidal (middle turbinate removal)

Transnasal direct

The operation is performed through one nostril. If the nasal cavity is very narrow and the passage of the endoscope and operating instruments is limited because of a septal deviation, septoplasty is performed first. After the middle and superior turbinates, the posterior region of the nasal septum, and the choanal arch have been identified, the ostium of the sphenoid sinus is probed with the seeker. To improve access, the superior turbinate is identified and removed with a through-cutting forceps. When the surgical access is very narrow, the posterior portion of the middle turbinate can also be removed with a microscissors.

The initial opening of the sphenoid sinus is made with a micro-Kerrison punch, beginning at the ostium. The sphenoidotomy is enlarged inferiorly and laterally while carefully avoiding or cauterizing the septal artery that crosses the anterior wall of the sphenoid sinus in that region. The 4-mm

0° endoscope is used for this step. This approach can be particularly useful for the following clivus lesions: CSF fistula, clivus meningocele, clivus mucocele, and bacterial or fungal infections that erode the sphenoid sinus and involve the clivus.

Transseptal

The transseptal approach was conceived to provide midline access to the sphenoid sinus region through the nasal septum, avoiding damage to the structures in the nasal cavity and avoiding the lateral wall of the sphenoid sinus and the nearby carotid artery and optic nerve. The transseptal approach has been particularly useful in accessing the clivus, sella, and parasellar regions because these are midline structures.

The surgeon first performs a submucoperichondrial and submucoperiosteal infiltration using lidocaine (2%) and epinephrine (1:100.000), producing a hydraulic dissection that facilitates surgical elevation. A vertical hemitransfixion incision is made at the caudal edge of the septal cartilage and septal flaps are elevated as in performing a septoplasty. The osseocartilaginous junction (septal cartilage, ethmoid plate, and vomer) is disarticulated using the suction elevator, preserving the uppermost part of the osseocartilaginous junction to avoid postoperative dorsal nasal saddling. The posterior attachment of the septum to the perpendicular lamina of the ethmoid is fractured. The posterior part of the septal bone, which obstructs access to the sphenoid rostrum, is resected using a Jansen-Middleton forceps. The mucoperiosteum of the anterior wall of the sphenoid sinus is elevated until the sinus ostia on both sides are visualized. At this point, the anterior wall of the sphenoid sinus is entirely exposed. The sphenoid rostrum and the anterior wall are then opened with a chisel and are enlarged with a micro-Kerrison punch or high-speed drill. The sphenoidotomy is made large enough to allow easy simultaneous introduction of a 4-mm endoscope and a surgical instrument.

Although the caudal hemitransfixion incision is useful when a simultaneous correction of a septal deviation is necessary, making the initial septal incision more posteriorly, closer to the rostrum of the sphenoid sinus, is often advantageous. Pituitary tumors and inverted papillomas occasionally recur in the sphenoid sinus, and in these situations a more posterior incision avoids repeated dissection of scarred septal flaps. For this procedures, a vertical transfixion incision is made 1.5 cm anterior to the sphenoid sinus ostium, joining a second horizontal incision 1 cm below the superior edge of the nasal septum. The mucoperiosteum of both sides can be removed or just retracted laterally, and the bony nasal septum is then removed. If a dural defect is present at the end of the procedure, the mucoperiosteal flap can be used in the dural repair.

The transseptal approach to the sphenoid sinus can be extended to access the sella, parasellar regions, petrous apex, clivus, and cavernous sinus.

*Transnasal with removal of the posterior part of the nasal septum
(two-nostril approach)*

The posterior part of the nasal septum can be removed to enlarge the operative field. The septal mucosa can be elevated and retracted on one or both sides and then replaced or removed at the end of the procedure. This modification permits two surgeons to work simultaneously, one through each nostril. The use of three or four instruments, including the endoscope, facilitates tumor removal and control of any intradural bleeding. It is also very helpful when removing large lesions in the posterior third of the nasal cavity, sphenoid sinus, clivus, sella, and parasellar regions (especially highly vascularized tumors), and is essential in cases with intradural extension.

*Transnasal direct combined with transethmoidal
(middle turbinate removal)*

When a larger operative field is desired, the transethmoidal approach may be combined with the direct transnasal approach. This combined approach is particularly useful for clivus chordoma, petrous apex lesions, and lesions that extend to the lateral recess of the sphenoid sinus.

First, an ethmoidectomy is performed beginning with the resection of the uncinate process and followed by resection of the ethmoid bulla and the remaining ethmoid cells. During the resection of the posterior ethmoid cells, the surgeon must correlate direct observation and intraoperative review of the CT scan to determine whether an Onodi cell is present, and if so, to understand its relationship to the optic canal and ICA.

The initial opening of the sphenoid sinus is made with a delicate curette or an atraumatic aspirator medially and inferiorly. The sphenoidotomy is then enlarged using a micro-Kerrison punch, incorporating the natural ostium into the opening.

Removal of the middle turbinate is usually necessary to create a single cavity between the nasal septum and the medial wall of the orbit. When an even larger surgical field is needed, bilateral ethmoidectomy and resection of both middle turbinates are performed. The middle turbinate mucoperiosteum can be used as a free graft to repair dural defects that were created by the lesion or its removal.

Transsphenoidal and transclival approaches to the cavernous sinus

Although anterior approaches offer a more direct anatomic approach to the structures beyond the clivus, the risks for CSF leakage and infection limit most of the previously mentioned approaches to extradural lesions, especially those that traverse a potentially unsterile operative field [12]. The major advantage of the midline transfacial approaches is the direct anterior surgical access through the large spaces of the nasal cavity, nasopharynx, oral cavity, and paranasal sinuses. However, these midline routes are restricted by critical neurovascular structures such as the ICA, optic nerve, cavernous sinus, cranial nerves, and orbital contents [16].

The transnasal endoscopic-assisted surgical technique begins by using one of the surgical approaches to the sphenoid sinus (transnasal direct, transethmoidal, or transseptal). A micro-Kerrison punch is used to obtain a wide opening of the anterior sphenoid sinus wall. The floor of the sella, the two carotid protuberances, the medial aspect of the optic canals, and the upper clivus are identified. The sinus mucosa that lines the clival area is reflected carefully, exposing the clival bone. The bone is initially removed using a drill system with a diamond burr and continued carefully with a micro-Kerrison punch if necessary (Fig. 4). The clival bone is usually removed as far as the floor of the sella superiorly, the foramen magnum inferiorly, and the bony canals of the sixth cranial nerves, the internal carotid arteries, and the occipital condyles laterally. This technique is used for extradural lesions (Fig. 5A, B). To obtain an intradural exposure, the external layer of the dura is first incised and the basilar venous plexus and cranial nerve VI are encountered. Bleeding in the plexus cannot be cauterized safely but usually can be controlled with small pieces of Surgicel. Large lesions often encroach on and obliterate much of the plexus, but if the lesion is not large or the plexus not completely compressed, profuse and intense bleeding can occur. Control of this bleeding requires judicious packing, time, patience, and experience.

The internal layer of the dura at the level of the middle and superior clivus must be opened with great care to avoid injury to the underlying basilar artery. Once the dura is opened and minor bleeding is stopped using bipolar coagulation, the endoscopes can finally be introduced carefully into the intradural space, and the major vessels of the posterior fossa (eg, basilar artery and branches; AICA; vertebral arteries; superior cerebellar and posterior

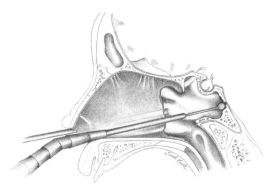

Fig. 4. Schematic drawing showing a modified transseptal approach to the posterior sphenoid sinus wall (clivus). A long handpiece with diamond burr is used to remove the bone of the upper clivus.

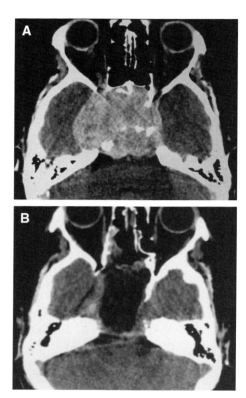

Fig. 5. (*A*) Preoperative axial CT of a patient who has an extradural clivus chordoma. (*B*) Postoperative axial CT of the patient seen in Fig. 5A after endoscopic resection of the extradural clivus chordoma.

cerebral arteries); the intradural course of cranial nerves III, IV, V, and VI; the brainstem; and the mammillary bodies can be identified. The cerebellopontine angle, cranial nerves VII through XII, and the retrosellar regions are best visualized using endoscopes of 30°, 45°, or 70° (Fig. 6).

Large dural defects at the clivus region are difficult to repair. We usually seal such defects with fat, fascia lata, and nasal septal mucoperiosteum/middle turbinate grafts. These grafts are kept in place with fibrin glue and pieces of Gelfoam (Pharmacia & Upjohn Company, Kalamazoo, Michigan). The nasal cavity is packed with Merocel (Medtronic Xomed, Jacksonville, Florida) for 3 to 5 days. A lumbar subarachnoid drain is not often necessary. Broad-spectrum antibiotics are used for 10 days.

The transsphenoidal transclival approach with removal of the posterior nasal septum has two main advantages: avoiding cerebral retraction and a decreased incidence of injury to the lower cranial nerves. In addition, the approach is direct without external incisions, is quick, and best preserves the anatomic structures. Although endoscopes do not allow a three-dimensional

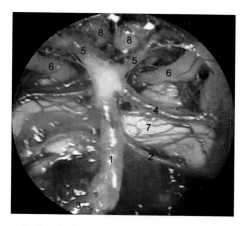

Fig. 6. Surgical endoscopic view during a transseptal transclival approach (1, basilar artery and branches; 2, AICA; 3, vertebral artery; 4, superior cerebellar artery; 5, posterior cerebral arteries; 6, intradural course of cranial nerve III; 7, brainstem; 8, mamillary bodies).

perspective, they provide a close view of the operative field from different angles. However, this technique requires the surgeon to work in a narrow operative field limited by critical neurovascular structures, such as internal carotid arteries; optic nerves; cavernous and basilar sinuses; and the pituitary gland. The risks for major intradural bleeding, CSF leakage, and meningitis must not be taken lightly. This technique is often used for clivus chordoma removal (Fig. 7A, B).

Transclival approach to the petrous apex

The transclival approach to the petrous apex can be useful for biopsy and drainage purposes. This type of surgical access can be particularly helpful in selected cases of cholesterol granuloma of the petrous apex because complete excision is unnecessary (Fig. 8A, B). Although surgical drainage is usually accomplished through the temporal bone, the transsphenoidal transclival endoscopic approach may be indicated when the lesion abuts the posterior and lateral wall of the sphenoid sinus. In these cases, an image guidance system can be very helpful, especially for precise identification of the ICA and optic nerve [17].

Repair of cerebrospinal fluid leaks and dural defects

CSF leakage can occur during any skull base procedure. The skull base surgeon must anticipate and identify intraoperative dural defects and be prepared to treat them as part of the planned surgical procedure. The same principles apply when CSF fistulas are repaired as a primary procedure.

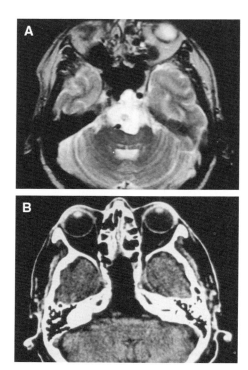

Fig. 7. (*A*) Preoperative axial MRI of a patient who has a clivus chordoma with intradural extension. (*B*) Postoperative axial CT of the same patient shown in Fig. 7A after endoscopic resection.

The surgical techniques for repairing a CSF fistula have the same principles, regardless of the location of the fistula: identifying the site of the fistula, and repairing it with a free mucoperiosteal graft from the inferior or middle turbinate or from the nasal septum. For large defects, we use a two-layer closure of fascia lata and mucoperiosteum, sealed with fibrin glue and covered with Gelfoam and nasal packing [18]. Synthetic material such as Duragen (Integra Life Sciences Corporation, Plainsboro, New Jersey) and Duraform (Codman, Raynham, Massachusetts) may also be used to help seal the fistulas. Lumbar subarachnoid drain should be initially avoided in cases of large defects because of the possibility for tension pneumocephalus. If a low-volume fistula appears a few days later, it may be treated with lumbar catheter placement alone.

Authors' experience

From 1995 to 2005, the authors endoscopically removed 36 lesions of the clivus region without an external approach. Not all of the lesions originated from the clivus; some arose from adjacent regions. The most frequent clivus

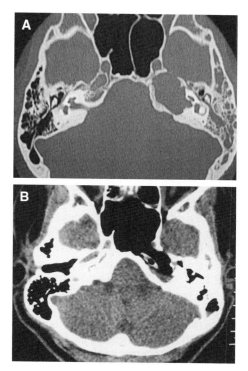

Fig. 8. (*A*) Axial CT of a cholesterol granuloma of the petrous apex. (The patient presented with left cranial nerve VII paralysis and left mixed hearing loss). (*B*) Postoperative CT of the same patient shown in Fig. 8A. (Note the apical communication into sphenoid sinus and presence of drainage catheter.)

lesions in our series were clivus chordoma; primary CSF fistulae; meningocele and meningoencephalocele; and clivus teratoma. Clivus-related lesions included angiofibroma, cholesterol granuloma of the petrous apex, and infection of the sphenoid sinus (Table 1).

Complications

Every clivus surgical procedure has potential complications. Prevention of the complications of transnasal endoscopic-assisted surgery of skull base begins with an adequate preoperative evaluation of the patient, including history of medication use and previous operations. High-resolution CT in coronal and axial projections with sagittal reconstruction, MRI, and sometimes angiography are essential in planning the procedure and executing it safely with the lowest possibility of complications.

Complications can be classified as *minor* or *major* according to severity, and as *immediate* or *delayed* according to time of appearance. Minor

Table 1
Frequency of clivus lesions operated through endoscopic transnasal approach (1995–2005)

Clival lesions	Number
Clivus chordoma	13
Cholesterol granuloma (petrous apex)	04
Cholesterol granuloma (clivus)	02
Primary CSF fistula	04
Traumatic CSF fistula	02
Clival meningocele	02
Intraclival mucocele	02
Fungal disease	04
Clivus teratoma	01
Malignant tumors	03

complications present little morbidity and do not compromise the life of the patient, although they may be annoying and troublesome. Most minor complications resolve with time and conservative treatment. However, major complications present significant morbidity and the possibility of mortality. Most orbital complications stem from direct injury to the optic nerve or the extraocular muscles, or from arterial or venous bleeding within the rigid bony orbit. These injuries can result in diplopia, hematoma, proptosis, decreased visual acuity, or blindness (which can be temporary or permanent). Blindness secondary to orbital hematoma can be reversible and mandates prompt hematoma evacuation to relieve the increased pressure compromising the blood supply to the retina or the optic nerve. Direct or indirect damage to the optic nerve usually occurs at the superolateral sphenoid sinus wall or in the posterior ethmoid cells.

Intracranial complications can result from direct injury to brain, cranial nerves, meninges, blood vessels, or venous sinuses. The resulting deficits reflect the loss of function of damaged structures in the case of brain and cranial nerves, the effects of loss of vascular supply to critical areas (stroke), or the mass effect of a resulting hematoma. Additionally, CSF leakage can cause symptoms directly and predispose to meningitis, and air entering the brain (pneumocephalus) can cause mass effect symptoms.

Bleeding is a risk in any surgical procedure, but seldom are so many important vessels susceptible to injury. The transnasal approaches visualize and place at risk the anterior and posterior ethmoid arteries; the sphenopalatine and maxillary arteries and their branches; the ICA; the anterior cerebral, basilar, and vertebral arteries and their branches; and the venous sinuses of the skull base (the cavernous sinus, basilar venous plexus, and the anterior intercavernous sinus).

Severe injuries of the ICA can be catastrophic and lethal. In cases of minor injuries, we recommend the following measures: 1) packing the sphenoid sinus and nose; 2) compressing the ICA in the neck; 3) temporarily lowering the blood pressure (hypotensive anesthesia); 4) blood transfusion as necessary; and 5) neurosurgical assistance. After controlling the bleeding, angiography is mandatory to evaluate the possibility of pseudo-aneurysm formation and the cross-circulation, because an occlusion of the ICA or stents may be needed.

The most frequent immediate complications are CSF leakage, intraoperative bleeding, orbital hematoma, brain injury, and intrasellar complications, which can include injuries of the diaphragma sella; arachnoid membrane; pituitary stalk; intra-arachnoid vascular structures; and the hypothalamus, optic nerve, and chiasm and their surrounding vessels. Injuries to cranial nerves III and VI are uncommon except in the transsphenoidal transclival approaches. Delayed complications include progressive loss of vision or smell, meningitis, bleeding, synechia, and infection. The surgeon must also be aware of the possibility of transitory or permanent endocrinologic complications that can result from manipulation, compression, or traction of the pituitary stalk. The surgeon must be able to diagnose acute anterior pituitary insufficiency and manage this condition, or have available appropriate consultants who can.

Postoperative care

The goal of surgical treatment is to assure complete removal of the disease, and the best possible functional result. A satisfactory postoperative result depends on appropriate operative technique and meticulous postoperative care.

Wide-spectrum antibiotics are given during the operation and for 10 days postoperatively. Adequate postoperative care of the operative site requires appropriate instrumentation, including 4-mm 0°, 45°, and 70° endoscopes; straight and curved atraumatic aspirators; and straight and curved microforceps.

We remove all packing 2 to 4 days after surgery (earlier for uncomplicated cases, but no longer than 4 days for extensive procedures or those with more aggressive diseases). The operative cavity is carefully suctioned and any residual bony fragments are removed. A second visit is scheduled between the 10th and 12th day after surgery and the operated cavity is again cleaned of crusts, granulation tissue, clots, and secretions. A third visit is scheduled between the third and fourth postoperative week. By then, the surgical cavity usually appears to be healing well. Image study is recommended 3 months after surgery to verify the postoperative status. CT or MRI is performed earlier if healing does not seem to be progressing satisfactorily or if complications are suspected.

Summary

Transnasal endoscopic-assisted techniques to the clivus region can be safe and effective. Endoscopic-assisted approaches provide improved visualization and are a superior alternative to open surgical approaches in most cases. Nevertheless, problems such as infection, CSF leakage, and difficulty controlling intradural bleeding still remain. Surgeons must always remember that, although high technology such as endoscopes, image-guided surgery systems, imaging studies, and advanced anesthetic drugs were essential for the development and improvement of the skull base surgery, the success of this type of surgery depends on perfect knowledge of the anatomy, intense endoscopic surgery training, and a multidisciplinary partnership.

References

[1] Stamm AC, Pignatari SSN. Transnasal endoscopic-assisted surgery of the skull base. In: Cummings CW, Flint PW, Harker LA, editors. Otolaryngology head neck surgery. 4th edition. Philadelphia: Elsevier Mosby; 2005. p. 3855–76.

[2] Crockard HA. The transoral approach to the base of the brain and upper cervical cord. Ann R Coll Surg Engl 1985;67:321–5.

[3] Draf W, Weber R, Keerl R. Endonasale chirurgie von tumoren der nasennebenhohlen und rhinobasis. Med Bild Dienst 1995;2:13–7.

[4] Harsh GR, Joseph MP, Swearingen B, et al. Anterior midline approaches to the central skull base. Clin Neurosurg 1996;43:15–43.

[5] Alfieri A, Jho HD. Endoscopic endonasal approach to the cavernous sinus. An anatomical study. Neurosurgery 2001;48:1–11.

[6] Jho HD. The expanding role of endoscopy in skull base surgery. Clin Neurosurg 2001;48: 278–305.

[7] Fujii K, Chambers SM, Rhoton AL Jr. Neurovascular relationship of the sphenoid sinus. A microsurgical study. J Neurosurg 1979;50:31–9.

[8] Lang J. Clinical Anatomy of the nose, nasal cavity and paranasal sinus. NY: Thieme; 1989.

[9] Siebert DR. Estudo anatômico de seios esfenoidais em brasileiros adultos [thesis]. São Paulo, Brazil: University of São Paulo; 1992.

[10] Jho HD, Ha HG. Endoscopic endonasal skull base surgery: part 3- the clivus and posterior fossa. Minim Invasive Neurosurg 2004;47(1):16–23.

[11] Zhou D, Patil AA, Rodriguez-Sierra J. Endoscopic neuroanatomy through the sphenoid sinus. Minim Invasive Neurosurg 2005;48:19–24.

[12] Puxeddu R, Lui MWM, Chandrasekar K, et al. Endoscopic-assisted transcolumellar approach to the clivus: an anatomical study. Laryngoscope 2002;112:1072–8.

[13] Stammberger H, Greistorfer K, Wolf G, et al. Surgical occlusion of cerebrospinal fistulas of the anterior skull base using intrathecal sodium fluorescein. Laryngorhinootologie 1997;76: 595–607.

[14] Lam SM, Huang C, Newman J, et al. Computer aided image guided endoscopic sinus surgery in unusual cases of sphenoid disease. Rhinology 2002;40:179–84.

[15] Gibbons M, Sillers MJ. Minimally invasive approaches to the sphenoid sinus. Otolaryngol Head Neck Surg 2002;126:635–41.

[16] Hitotsumatsu T, Matsushima T, Rhoton AL. Surgical anatomy of the midface and the midline skull base. Oper Tech Neurosurg 1999;2:160–80.

[17] Stamm AC, Pignatari SSN, Sebusiani BB, et al. Endoscopic surgery of the paranasal sinuses and skull base by using the image guided system. Rev Bras Otorrinolaringol 2002;68:502–9.

[18] Stamm AC. Micro-endoscopic surgery of the paranasal sinuses. In: Stamm AC, Draf W, editors. Micro-endoscopic surgery of the paranasal sinuses and the skull base. Heildelberg: Springer; 2000. p. 201–36.

ELSEVIER
SAUNDERS

Otolaryngol Clin N Am
39 (2006) 657–660

OTOLARYNGOLOGIC
CLINICS
OF NORTH AMERICA

Index

Note: Page numbers of article titles are in **boldface** type.

0030-6665/06/$ - see front matter © 2006 Elsevier Inc. All rights reserved.
doi:10.1016/S0030-6665(06)00061-2